The Making of a
Joyful Mother

The Making of a Joyful Mother

A Spiritual Journey for Women Experiencing Infertility

Kimberly Webb

iUniverse, Inc.

New York Lincoln Shanghai

The Making of a Joyful Mother
A Spiritual Journey for Women Experiencing Infertility

iUniverse books may be ordered through booksellers or by contacting:

iUniverse
2021 Pine Lake Road, Suite 100
Lincoln, NE 68512
www.iuniverse.com
1-800-Authors (1-800-288-4677)

Scripture taken from the NEW AMERICAN STANDARD BIBLE®
Copyright © 1960, 1962, 1963, 1968, 1971, 1972, 1973, 1975, 1977, 1994 by the Lockman Foundation. Used by permission.

Visit our Web site at www.kimberlywebb.org

ISBN-13: 978-0-595-39449-4 (pbk)
ISBN-13: 978-0-595-83846-2 (ebk)
ISBN-10: 0-595-39449-3 (pbk)
ISBN-10: 0-595-83846-4 (ebk)

Printed in the United States of America

Psalms 113:9

*"He makes the barren women abide in the house,
as a joyful mother of children. Praise the Lord"*

Contents

Acknowledgments

The completion of this book has been a long, but rewarding process. Although it has been a challenging journey, I must thank the many people who pushed me forward toward my dreams.

First, I have to thank God for giving me a purpose and having patience with me when I did not want to fulfill my purpose. Without Jesus Christ in my life, constantly nudging and pushing me forward, I truly don't know where I would be. Thank you for continuing to love me in spite of me. Thank you for giving me Kendal.

I want to give special thanks to my husband, Steven for his tireless efforts in motivating me to finish this work. Steven helped me edit this book and is also responsible for designing my website, and my business cards. But, above all, he is responsible for loving me and pushing me forward when I wanted to quit so many times. Thank you Steven for believing in me, when sometimes, I did not believe in myself. I love you so much!

Thanks to my parents for loving me enough to introduce me to Jesus Christ. Thank you for instilling confidence in me to know that I can do all things through Christ. Thanks for you love and support of this project and everything that I put my hands to. Thanks for your constant prayers.

Thanks to my sister, Kelli and her husband Malachi Nance for your loving support during this project.

Thanks to my grandmother, MeMe who constantly encouraged me to follow God's plan for my life no matter what anyone else says.

Thanks to my uncle, John Thacker, for convincing me to pursue my dreams, buy a laptop computer and start writing this book. In addition, thank you for listening to me and providing me with sound advice.

Thanks to Pastor Anthony T. Evans, founder of The Urban Alternative and pastor of Oak Cliff Bible Fellowship and my church family in Dallas, Texas, for providing my biblical training and truly bringing the Word of God to life for my husband and me.

Thanks to Pastors Gordon and Derozette Banks, for allowing God to use your prophetic gifts to minister over Steven and me. Thank you Pastor Gordon for using your anointing to pray over us during our barren season and allowing us to piggyback on your faith in God for our miracle. Thank you Pastor Derozette for prophesying over me and watching "your child" fulfill her calling.

Thanks to Pastor Mike Hayes, pastor of Covenant Church and my church family in Carrollton, Texas, for creating an atmosphere of praise and worship that taught me about the gifts of the Holy Spirit.

Thanks to Dr. Robert Milstein, who performed so many surgeries on me. Thank you for receiving and applying the knowledge that God gave you concerning my body.

Thanks to our dear friends, Ferlonzo and Osha Knott, for the encouraging and uplifting conversations that we have on every Sunday afternoon. You are both sister and brother to Steven and me. We love you both and can't wait to see where God is going to take you in your ministry.

Thanks to Don Carter, my professor at Covenant Training Institute, for seeing something in me that I did not see in myself. For directing, pushing and guiding me to complete this work and launch my business. In a loving way, you were tough on me—but I needed that.

Thanks to Karen Rodgers for being a living example of a loving, protective, and caring mother who sacrificed daily for her child. Bravo, you did an outstanding job in raising Tiffany. Thank you for just allowing me to watch and learn.

Thanks to Tracy Dubose, my lifelong friend, for always thinking "out-of-the-box." Thank you for not only teaching me to dream, but helping me to live the dream.

Thanks to William and Grenna Rollings for helping me walk through this writing publishing journey. Be inspired William, your book is next!

Thank to Patryce Curtis, my Howard University sister. It's been a lot of years and even more memories. I treasure your friendship. Thanks so much for remaining true.

Thanks to my Critique Group:

Kiva Oby—my precious little sister, thank you for being such a good friend who encourages me and is not afraid to speak the truth. Thank you for not only reviewing my book proposal, but for listening to my countless concerns and helping me to see the brighter side of life. You are always in my corner.

Jennifer Peete—thank you for taking your time to edit my book proposal and for providing your marketing expertise. I am thankful for our new found friendship.

Corlis Webb—my sister-in-law, for your prophetic gift and allowing God to use you when I needed to hear from Him most. Thank you for reviewing my book proposal.

Thanks to Deborah Bolden, aka "Dr. D," for your countless hours of advice and encouragement. Thank you for making sure that I always had everything I needed. You never let me give up.

Thanks to Tia Texada, from the day I met you, you have been constant encouragement to me. You are compassionate, transparent and real.

Thanks to Barbara Bostic, for providing professional editing services and positive feedback on the book. Thanks so much for the quick turnaround time and the special comments you provided.

Thanks to the Essence Book Club in Dallas, Texas for encouraging me during this endeavor. (Nikole Allen, Kiva Oby, Mary Hayes, Sonya Jackson, and Sharniqua Glaspie)

Thanks to Jeff Crilley who encouraged to get this book ASAP and provided tips on media coverage and publishing.

Special Thanks to Pastor George & Sister Alma Pryor, Pastor Ricky Rush, Erie Jr. Land, LaMaron and Rosalyn Pryor, Dr. Paul & Janetta Webb, Eldora and Gene Humphrey, my Covenant Life Team, Pastor Josef Rasheed, Joe and Ramona Bailey, Varn and Earma Brown, Theresa Jackson at the Promise Shoppe, Ava Howard, Rebecca Emerson, James Huckaby, Renissa Wade, Dr. Alvin Thornton—Howard University, Darren Allen, Roxanne Ballard, Scarlet Bayard, Adrienne Irvin, Monica Hayes, Ron and Sandra Eaton, Carl and Trishell Seymore, Ward and Ruth Griffin, Steve and Cynthia Smith, Tim and Tiffany Jones, Mary Ellen Hicks, Deborah Peoples, Kathleen Hicks, Chaney and Whitney Peoples, Drenea Mack, Pamela Gasaway, Sherri and Norm Williams, and Ray and Rosemarie Williams.

If I have forgotten anyone, please forgive me. But as you can see, the list is quite long and rivals an Academy Award acceptance speech, so please accept my humble apologies.

My Prayer

Father, I thank You for giving me the opportunity to pour my struggle into a book to help women facing emptiness, fear, physical let down, emotional inadequacy, longsuffering, anxiety and pain in the area of conception and pregnancy.

I pray that you will reveal to us your definition of whom You are and who we are in relation to You. Lord Jesus, help us to examine and determine why we want to have and raise children. Give us wisdom and teach us to match our desire with Your will.

Be with us Lord, as we wait to hear from You. Hold us up and have mercy on us, when we continue to demonstrate a lack of faith. Be our comforter, and pick us up when our cycles are late and disappointment sets in. Remind us of Your presence in our lives, and give us Your grace when our womb is empty and cold and we feel deserted and alone. Grant us peace as we learn Your direction for our lives and lean to You for our destiny. Father, let us show You the joy we have for our deliverance. Let us give You all the glory for our beautiful, healthy babies that You will bless us with! Thank You Lord, in advance, for Your mercy and Your patience with us. Bless each reader of this book with unbeatable faith.

I pray that women will read and take heed that You are the Almighty God, Creator of heaven and earth and all its inhabitants. Touch their bodies, heal emotional and internal wounds. Prepare their hearts and minds for motherhood. Above all, may this experience bring them closer to You. Lord, make these women fertile with your word. I pray that every woman reading this book will become the joyful mother You created them to be!

In the matchless name of Jesus Christ,
Amen

Introduction

Giving birth to a child is the most basic function of a woman. When her body is unable to produce, it causes her to question herself, her life, her husband, and eventually her God. Many women have struggled with infertility for years and believe their window of opportunity has passed, or they've experienced serious medical conditions and deem that these conditions are blocking their fertility. Yet, others believe that God must be punishing them for something they've done in their past. While these issues are valid concerns, I want you to know that God is not willing to birth a new creation out of us until He can birth a greater creation in us. Until God is free to change some things inside our hearts and minds, we will forever live stagnant and defeated lives.

As a woman who struggled for years with medical problems including fibroid tumors, endometriosis, irregular periods, miscarriages and even a tubal pregnancy, I am all too familiar with the trial of infertility. I've had first-hand experience with the physical pain and emotional strain that this struggle causes. But I want you to know; God has seen me through all the pain and blessed me on the other side of the trial.

The Bible says that He has overcome the world and all things are possible through Him—that includes opening your womb and removing any medical roadblocks. If we can truly believe this, we must believe that God has a greater purpose for what we're experiencing.

This book is meant to challenge you to look past your empty belly and focus your attention on why God is using this trial to get your attention. As you read this book, treat it just like you enrolled in a course at school, except this course is not about math or history. This course is called "Trust God 101."

I

The Daughter's Struggle with Infertility

1

Day of Dependence

Isaiah 22:11 "...but you did not depend on Him who made it, nor did you take into consideration Him who planned it long ago."

Steven comes home from work and is extremely excited about a co-worker of his who just had a baby. He wants to go and visit her at the hospital. I was friends with her as well, so I agree. We arrive at the hospital to visit our friend and she is holding her new little angel. We step beside her bed and Steven says, "Can I hold her." Our friend says, "Sure." He picks up this sweet little girl and immediately he's swept away. As we are driving home, Steven says to me, "Kim, when do you think we can start trying to have a baby." I reply, "Well, I guess we can start trying now." Steven was elated. As soon as I finished my statement, he decided that he wanted a little boy; because he didn't think he could handle a little girl. He was afraid that he would love a girl too much; whereas with a boy, he could be rough and tough.

As you can see, in the beginning my husband and I did not depend on God for a child. We simply decided that it was time for us to have a family and pursued that goal. It wasn't until some time much later that we determined we needed God in this area. We assumed, like everyone else, having a baby was a natural and basic process; all we had to do is decide when we wanted to have a baby and just have one. Sure, I had heard of infertility, but I thought *that* only happened to a small segment of the community. Frankly, I did not believe that I was in that small segment. It was not until much later that I found out that I was one of more than 6.1 million women in the United States who suffer from this epidemic. So don't ever feel like you are alone in this battle, you are not. For me, this was a real wakeup call. I had prayed and believed God for other areas in my life, I never thought I needed to bring this area to God. Unintentionally, I was functioning completely independent of God. Again, I assumed that conception was an event that would just happen. The sooner I realized that I could not do this on my own without God, the better off I was.

Interestingly enough, we can all learn a few things from babies. You see, babies quickly realize that they depend on their caregivers (mothers, fathers or babysitters) to meet their needs and crying out for help works because someone comes to give them exactly what they need. Smarter than we think, babies have processed three concepts: the realization of their limitations as babies; crying is their call for help; and the faith to believe someone will come.

First, the baby realizes his dependence on others because of his limitations. He feels the frustration of not being able to get his food, change his diaper, turn on the light, or calm his fears. The second concept is this noise of crying which gets the caregivers attention. Every time the baby cries, the caregiver is alerted that something is wrong with the baby and he needs something. *The Bible states in Exodus 22:23, "If he does cry out to Me, I will surely hear his cry."* Isn't it amazing that we are like babies in so many ways. When life hurts us and we are scared, we cry out and want someone to make us all better. Unfortunately, sometimes we cry out to others, who can only listen and sympathize with our problems, when we should cry out to God who answers our prayers and supplies our needs. God sees us as His babies who need his help and He is willing and ready to help us.

In essence, babies recognize that as there are some things that they cannot do on their own. But instead of trying to do it themselves, they learn to look toward someone else who has the ability and the means to help them. *The Bible states in Isaiah 41:10, "Do not fear for I am with you; do not anxiously look about you, for I am your God. I will strengthen you, surely I will help you, surely I will uphold you with My righteous right hand."* When we accept our position as God's children and realize that we can't do it all ourselves, then our Heavenly Father steps in and makes our life easier to live.

The third concept a baby uses is faith. Babies use their voices to ask their mother to meet their need. They rely on the faith that Mommy will be able to meet that need.

The Bible states in Mark 11:23-24, "Truly I say to you, whoever says to this mountain, be taken up and cast into the sea, and does not doubt in his heart, but believes that what he says is going to happen, it will be granted him. Therefore I say to you, all things for which you pray and ask, believe that you have received them and they will be granted him."

God always tests us in the areas where our faith is the weakest. I've been a Christian for a long time, and truly believe that prayer is power and that God can change any circumstance. I am not sure why I didn't consult God in the beginning. However, I quickly learned through this trial that we must bring everything to God in prayer even things we take for granted. Because it is when we take those things for granted that we are acting independently of God. I questioned why I was not able to get pregnant? I performed all my Christian responsibilities and still nothing. Somehow, I had it all wrong.

God was not going to bless my womb just because I thought I was a good Christian. This was not about "you do this for me and I'll do that for you." The basis of Christianity is faith in God and dependence on Him. So I was looking at my situation all wrong. As I pondered my situation and questioned my thinking, it occurred to me that I needed to be dependent on Him; but, I wasn't dependent on Him. Instead of letting go and letting God, I continued to feel the need to help God out. Maybe if I could relax more or maybe if I elevated my legs after sex, I could conceive. But God was not interested in my tricks, He wanted me to be dependent on Him; and in order to be dependent, I had to first be content. God was trying to get me to a place of peace. The fact of the matter was that my husband and I had been trying to conceive for several years. In addition to that, I had already had a miscarriage and four surgeries in two years to correct internal female problems. The OB/GYN practice had four partners and three of the four had operated on me at least once and one doctor twice. I was dependent on God for everything else, except a healthy, beautiful baby.

One of the great things about God is that He does not leave us alone to figure things out on our own. He hears our cry when we recognize our position and increases our faith in the area where we are weak. If you will walk with God through your trial, continue to trust in Him and depend on Him to guide you; He will send you little glimmers of hope. A glimmer is a faint, unsteady light that is sometimes quick and fleeting. Fortunately for us, with life's constant struggles, God frequently provides us with these glimmers. I have found in my journey that God provides glimmers of hope when we least expect them and from people we least expect. However, some of my glimmers of hope have been from encouragement and some from prophecy.

Prophecy is the ability to proclaim new revelation or predict the future by the influence of divine guidance which is from God. For some of us, prophecy is a foreign term. Even in most churches, prophecy is not talked about or recognized. Prophecy is listed as one of the spiritual gifts given to Christians. I can say for myself, I had heard of prophecy, but I did not have any real knowledge of it nor did I think it was relevant to me or my situation. But let me tell you, prophecy is alive and well. It is not a gift that is to be taken lightly. Not everyone has the gift of prophecy, just like not everyone has the gift of healing. During the time I was trying to conceive and wanted a baby so desperately, I had three people prophesy to me.

The first glimmer of hope was in the form of encouragement from a friend that went to school with my husband. At the time, she was pregnant with her first child. She had encouraged me and told me that I was going to be pregnant, too. God was going to give me a baby. She told me of a book that she read and walked me to the bookstore, to purchase it. I bought the book, but it really did not address what I was going through. It focused more on actually giving birth not on conceiving. I remember her words though; she was so sure that God was going to answer my prayer. Later, I talked to my husband and he said even though the book did not help much, she was reassuring God's promises for us.

The second glimmer of hope was a prophetic word that came during Christmas. I always host Christmas dinner at my house while my family and friends come, eat and fellowship with us. I was sitting on the couch talking to a good friend of mine who happens to be a nurse. We were discussing the prognosis of my most recent surgery and my chances of having a baby. As we were talking, my brother-in-law's fiancée asked to speak with me in private, immediately. There were a lot of people in the house, so I suggested we go upstairs where it was quiet. We quickly went upstairs to the room I had chosen for our baby. I didn't know what she wanted to talk about; I just knew she was in a hurry to tell me something. She started off by saying, "I know this sounds crazy, but I was praying last week and God told me I would meet someone who was trying to have a baby." I didn't say anything, I just listened. She said, "He wants me to tell you that you are going to have a baby." The intellectual side of me would have quickly dismissed her, but her will and words were so strong. She said "when I first prayed and received this from God, I did not know who or how I would meet this person and tell them this news." She continued by saying, "God is so miraculous because He sent me here just to give you this message, I know God is going to bless your womb and you will give birth to a baby." Afterwards, she held my hand and touched my belly and prayed for me. As she was talking to me, it was as if God were talking to me right through her. It was the most unusual feeling, but it was also a calming feeling. Her presence was unyielding and you could tell she had faith as strong as an oak tree. Now realize, this was my first time to meet this young lady. I knew nothing about her except for her name and that she was engaged to my brother-in-law. That's all I knew about her.

The entire time she had been at my house, she had been friendly, but extremely quiet. However, I quickly found out that she was a Christian and she was not quiet about that. So we had a common link.

My third glimmer of hope was also a prophetic word from one of the associate ministers at our church. We had just completed new member orientation. Upon meeting the pastor, he asked us, if we had any children. Isn't it funny, when it's something you don't have, everyone always ask if you have it? My head dropped down and tears rolled down my face as my husband responded that we did not have any children. The pastor looked at me and inquired as to what was wrong. I explained all of the problems and complications that I had; and now these problems were causing us not to conceive or carry a baby to full term. He listened and looked at both of us with all the boldness and wisdom of an old man and said, "You will have a baby, I can look at you and see that you will give birth to a baby. God is going to do this." He looked at me as if he were looking straight through me to my soul. I looked at my husband and my husband looked back at the pastor. He explained that he knew of others that had similar problems, but trusted in God and God answered their prayers. But he looked at me with a glaring look, he said, "In six to seven months, you are going to come to me and tell me you are pregnant and I am going to already know. Before you tell me, I'll know; and we are going to praise God for His blessing and provision." This happened in late January. By late June, I was pregnant. *In 2 Peter 1:20-21, the Bible states, "but you know this first of all that no prophecy of scripture is a matter of one's own interpretation, for no prophecy was ever made by an act of human will, but men moved by the Holy Spirit spoke from God".* This scripture is very important. Everyone does not have the spiritual gift of prophecy, so you must be careful of those who think they have the gift and are instead advising you by what they think and not what they hear from God. I believe that God sent me these glimmers of hope because I was depending on Him and Him alone.

Sarah's Independence

Independence is a dangerous way to live your life. Independent people believe "If I really want something done, I have to do it myself." Independent people are strong, confident and assertive; and these can be perceived as good qualities until they are utilized in conflict with God. These are the qualities I exhibited early on my journey with infertility, however these characteristics must take a back seat and dependence must step in.

There are two ways you demonstrate your independence from God: **self-reliance,** meaning you rely only on yourself—developing your own plan and executing it your own way; the second is one I have termed "**self-glorification.**" Self-glorification is making decisions and plans that solely glorify you.

In the book of Genesis, Chapter 16, there is a story about a married couple named Abram and Sarai, their names were later changed to Abraham and Sarah. Sarah was considered barren and unable to conceive children. The Bible states that Sarah waited longer than 40 to 50 years for God to bless her womb, which is an extended length of time. During this time, God made a covenant with Abraham calling him to be the father of many nations. We know that both Abraham and Sarah wondered how God was going to perform this miracle with a man and woman who were both very old. The Bible does not talk about Sarah's faith in God, but let's assume Sarah had exercised her faith over and over and prayed constantly for a child; and God was silent. Sarah does state in *Genesis 16:2, "Now behold the Lord has prevented me from bearing children."*

In addition to this, Sarah probably said, "Enough is enough, I am already way past my child bearing years and every man needs a son to carry on the family name. Besides, God made a covenant with Abraham to make him a father of many nations." She decided that since God had prevented her from bearing children, she would find another way to provide Abraham with a son. Aren't we all a little like Sarah sometimes? We get frustrated with or impatient waiting for God's answer or lack of an answer to our prayers; and we decide to take matters into our own hands. We act in self-reliance like Sarah by developing and executing our own plans.

After many years of marriage and many efforts to conceive, Sarah sent Abraham to her maidservant Hagar for the purpose of having sex with Abraham and conceiving a child. Like every good man, Abraham did as he was told and had sex with Hagar; and Hagar conceived a son. The Bible says Abraham was 86 years old when Hagar gave birth to their son Ishmael.

Sarah celebrated her success. After all, her husband needed a son to fulfill the covenant and she had devised a way to make it happen. Her plan had worked; and she was a mother at last. Unexpectedly for her, the plan back-fired. As a result of this conception, Hagar despised Sarah and caused major problems in their home. This presented Sarah with an even bigger problem than the one she had when she started. It's amazing how we can develop a seemingly good plan to solve our problems, but for some reason, it fails to work out. Many times, we get it confused. We think that God may need or actually want us to help Him out. But dependency on God means that we take all our decisions and actions to Him first. Then we wait for His decision.

Sarah was independent. She believed that she had waited on God long enough and now it was time to act. She was getting old and feared that her biological clock had already stopped ticking; or maybe she thought God had forgotten about her and her prayer request. Do you think Sarah consulted with God before making the decision to give Hagar to Abraham? Absolutely, not. Realizing her error, she attempted to correct the problem by asking Abraham to make Hagar one of his wives—that still didn't work.

Using our own independent judgment can get us into trouble. Basically, being independent can create more problems and/or compound the ones we already have. Because we are human and prone to sin, we always want to think our way through life. When we're unable to come up with a viable solution, then we consult others. We don't consult God until the end, when we're ready to give up. God allows us to have this independent mindset because He knows it will eventually drive us back to Him.

I wonder what would happen if we actually started with a mindset seeking God first. How would our lives be different? *The Bible says in Matthew 7:33, "Seek first His kingdom and His righteousness and all these things will be added to you."* I'm sure that many of us are dealing with situations concerning our marriages, finances and health conditions that we believe shouldn't exist for us. Most of our problems are because we have chosen to go it alone, independent of God. After we fail and find ourselves in a mess, then we ask for God to rescue us.

Sarah was like that. She didn't plan on Hagar's attitude toward her. She didn't think her maidservant would turn on her, but look what happened. Instead of having Abraham and Sarah, now we have Abraham, Sarah, Hagar, and Ishmael. God had given Abraham a promise that he would be a father of many nations. But instead of having faith that God would manifest His promise, Sarah now has to contend with a second wife and a stepson.

Hannah's Dependence

Now that we have explored a life independent of God, let's explore a life dependent on God. Dependent people recognize their limitations and rely on God for everything. There are three ways that you demonstrate your dependence on God, they are: 1) you show a total reliance on God; 2) you are open to His plan for your life; and 3) your goal is to glorify Him. There is a story in the Bible (1 Samuel), where a young woman named Hannah marries a man named Elkanah. Hannah was barren. In that day, if your first wife bore no children, then you could marry a second wife. And Elkanah did, he married Peninnah.

Peninnah provoked Hannah by making fun of her inability to bear children. Of course, Hannah was irritated by this and it started to show. Many of us know how Hannah felt. Maybe no one is making fun of your situation, but you are saddened because God has not blessed you with a child, yet. The Bible says that Peninnah continued this activity year after year. At one point, Hannah began to cry and eventually stopped eating. She had allowed herself to be tormented so much by Peninnah that it drove her into a bout with depression.

But in her distress, Hannah prayed to the Lord as she wept. 1 Samuel 1:11 says, *"She made a vow and said, O Lord of hosts, if you will indeed look on the affliction of your maidservant and remember me and not forget your maidservant, but will give your maidservant a son, then I will give him to the Lord all the days of his life, and a razor shall never come on his head."* Hannah was relying on God. She did not fight back or use evil words toward Peninnah; she just prayed because she knew that God was the only one that could help her. Look at her prayer, she says "Lord, look on my affliction and remember me, don't forget me, remember me."

How many of us need God to remember us? The Bible says that she poured out her spirit. She prayed so hard that her husband thought she was drunk with wine, but she wasn't. She was serious with God and she didn't care who saw her. Some of us really need to get serious with God. We can't pray this prayer because we are not where Hannah was with her faith; and we have not been serious with God. When was the last time you poured your spirit out to God about having a baby? When was the last time you poured your spirit out to God about any issue? We don't ever need God to forget us. We need Him to remember us. Hannah relied on her God to pour out His favor upon her. Look at what else she said, *"But if you will give me a son, I will give him back to you."* Hannah was specific about what she wanted. She wanted a son. But

Hannah was open to God's plan for that son. The Bible says in *Luke 11:10*, *"for everyone who asks receives."* Have you asked God for what you want? If not, then I guess the question is "Why?"

The last sign of dependence is when you are more interested in glorifying Christ than you are in glorifying yourself. Hannah wanted a baby, but she also wanted to glorify God by giving her son back to the Lord. The Bible says that *"God remembered Hannah, and she conceived and gave birth to a son, Samuel, later a great king* (1 Samuel 1:19)."

Hannah didn't have a plan, she just had a God. Notice that Hannah did not follow Sarah's lead. She didn't try to devise a plan to get herself a baby. No, Hannah just waited and petitioned the Lord to remember her. And look at what Hannah says at the end, *"I will give him back to you Lord."* Do you have a plan to give your baby back to the Lord? Not that your child needs to become a preacher or a priest, but you need to make a commitment to raise your child to know the words and the ways of God.

Make this your prayer:

Dear Lord,

I come to you acknowledging that you are Lord over all my life. I repent from asserting my independence separate and apart from you. I am sorry; please forgive me for my actions. I am dependent upon you for everything, even little things I take for granted. Reveal areas in my life that I have acted independent of you. I have been independent for so long, please show me how to be dependent on you. I love you and want to glorify you. I am totally dependent on you to bring about this blessing of a child from my womb. I am no longer relying on others' advice; it's just you and me. Please give me a child so that I can give him back to you to be used by you as you please. Please speak to me and answer my prayers.

Your Daughter

In Jesus' Name,

Amen

2

Desire vs. God's Design

Psalms 37:4 "Delight yourself in the Lord; and
He will give you the desires of your heart."

Kim arrives just in time to meet her friend Susan for lunch. She greets Susan with a hug as they sit down and read the menu. Everything looks so good. Kim orders a chicken salad and Susan orders the same. Susan asks, "So, what's new? How's work and Steven?" Kim answers by saying, "Everything is fine, except Steven is ready to have a baby." She asks, "How do you feel about that?" Kim replies, "I'm Ok with it."

Then, Susan asked a question that neither Kim nor Steven had ever talked about. She asked, "Why do you want to have a baby?" Kim replied, "Well, we've been married for two years now, it's time. Besides, I would love to have a little baby to cuddle and love." Again, Susan questioned, "That's why you want a baby?"

Kim said, "Well, yes. Why do you want to have a baby?"

She stated, "I didn't say that I did. Frankly, I'm not sure that I want to. But if I did, I would at least have a decent reason for wanting a baby." This question continued to plague Kim for days. Why did she want a baby?

If you're reading this book, then most likely you have a desire to have a baby. But, why do you want a baby? Are your reasons for wanting a baby selfish or do you want to follow God's word to be "fruitful and multiply"? What about once He blesses you with a baby, are you going to make sure that the baby knows and loves God? Is your desire to have the baby for you or do you plan for the baby to have a purpose and be a vital part of God's kingdom?

Could your motives be for self-identity? Will having a child make you feel better about yourself? Maybe you were not loved as a child, or as a teen, or even as a wife. This lack of love has caused you to doubt and question whether you could even love yourself. Perhaps, if you could just have a baby, everything would fall into place. My friends, that is wrong thinking.

A baby can love you, but it cannot be held responsible for providing your emotional well-being. Children are lovable and sweet, but oftentimes they are not able to give the kind of love you need. Initially, they require feeding every 2-3 hours, constant diaper changes and nurturing. At such an early age, their only goal in life is to have their physical and emotional needs met. It would be completely unfair to place this burden on a baby who knows nothing about what you are feeling. Instead of waiting on a child to provide this kind of love for you, begin working on yourself.

Ask yourself, "Do I love me?" If the answer is "NO," find out why. Why don't you love yourself? What about you don't you love? Is it your appearance, your past, your career? Examine yourself. And after taking this introspective look at your motives, write these things down and title it "Me."

ME

Things I don't love about me	Ways I can change things I do not love about me	Scripture reference
Low self esteem	Begin to believe in myself regardless of how I feel or what others have told me in the past.	"I can do all things through Christ who strengthens me"

Maybe your issue is not about your love for yourself. Maybe you love yourself and you want a baby for other reasons. Perhaps the conflict rests between you and your husband. Is there a bond between you and your husband? Do you love him fully and completely? Or, is this baby going to solve the vast distance that lies between the two of you?

It's great to want a baby from a beautiful union of husband and wife, but if there is marital discord and you have not been able to conceive, God may decide that you need to wait. God's design may involve some changes to make your marriage harmonious. God could believe that in order for Him to bless you with a gift from heaven, He must first deal with your mess that the two of you have created here on earth, your marriage. Are you saving the love you should be lavishing on your husband for your new baby? If so, that is wrong in the sight of God and He is not pleased with your actions. In marriage, a husband and wife become one. If that oneness is really two-ness, then God sees the split; and He may decide not to bless that union until He sees oneness. I'm not saying that is why you are not pregnant, but this is an area where you want to make sure that you are in line with God's word. If your marriage is a façade, God sees the lie you live daily. Philippians 2:3 is summarized: To be united we must do nothing for selfish ambition, but regard one another as more important than ourselves. God wants our marriage to be a harmonious union where each spouse seeks to serve the needs of the mate above his/her own.

As Christians, we also believe that God gives us the desires of our heart. However, our desire may be different from God's design. God's design includes His timing and His perfect will for our lives. Sometimes, God's design matches our desires and sometimes it doesn't. In this chapter, we will examine the story of Rachel and Leah, analyzing their desires for wanting a baby and ours as well. We'll see how those desires fit into God's design for our lives.

In Genesis chapters 29-30, there is an interesting story about a man named Jacob who fell in love with a young lady named Rachel. Jacob asked Rachel's father Laban for her hand in marriage in exchange for his working for Laban seven years. Jacob worked seven years to earn Rachel's hand in marriage. Now Jacob was known as a trickster, as he tricked and schemed his way through life. Laban knew this to be true and decided to play a trick of his own. After seven years, instead of giving his daughter Rachel to Jacob, he decided to offer his oldest daughter, Leah. In those days, a woman's head and most of her face were covered. So of course, at the wedding, Jacob thought he was marrying Rachel, when in reality, he was marrying Leah. Of course, when Jacob found this out, he was quite angry. Cleverly, Laban worked another deal with Jacob, allowing Jacob to work an additional seven years in order to earn the hand of

Rachel. Long story short, Jacob agreed to the deal and worked seven more years to marry Rachel.

There were vast differences between the two sisters Rachel and Leah. First of all, Leah was the oldest daughter and the Bible describes her as not very attractive, unloved by Jacob, but very fertile. Rachel on the other hand had a good life; she was attractive, younger, but infertile. Jacob openly expressed his love for Rachel more. After both of the sisters were married to Jacob, Leah began to conceive babies and Rachel became jealous because she had not conceived. The Bible says in *Genesis 29:31, "Now the Lord saw that Leah was unloved, and He opened her womb, but Rachel was barren."* Rachel even blamed Jacob for her lack of conception. In *Gen. 30:1-2, Rachel says, "Give me children or else I die." Jacob's anger burned against Rachel and he said, "Am I in the place of God, who has withheld from you the fruit of the womb?"* Jacob pointed Rachel back to God. Rachel loved Jacob and wanted desperately to give him an heir. Since Rachel could not conceive herself, she honored her love and commitment to him by giving him her maid-servant Bilhah. Through Bilhah, Jacob would receive a son and heir from Rachel. Seeing what Rachel had done, Leah also gave her maid-servant to Jacob. In total, Leah bore Jacob six sons and one daughter…Then the Bible says that God remembered Rachel, her prayers and her commitment to her husband. God gave heed to her, opened her womb and she bore a son.

Let's examine each sister's desires regarding conceiving a child:

Leah's Desire

Leah desired to gain the love her husband. Leah gave birth to a son on three occasions, and each time she believed that her husband, Jacob would love her and become attached to her.

God's Design for Leah

In the *Gen. 29:31*, it states, *"Now the Lord saw that Leah was unloved and He opened her womb, but Rachel was barren."* The Bible doesn't go into great detail about Leah's life growing up, but I believe her life was probably not very pleasant. Unlike Rachel, Leah was not very attractive and likely suffered ridicule all her life. Remember, her father had to trick Jacob into marrying her. God felt compassion for her.

Her desire was to have children in order to make her husband love her, but her plan had failed and she was left again unloved. Leah delivers her fourth son and states, *"This time, I will praise the Lord."* God had to show Leah that desiring the love of her husband to fulfill her was not His design. God showed Leah the only way to have true fulfillment was through God. Upon understanding that, she began to praise Him for it.

Rachel's Desire

Rachel desired to have children for her husband and to compete with her very fertile sister, Leah.

God's Design for Rachel

God wanted to stop Rachel from competing with her sister and remove her jealousy.

We are told that Rachel was beautiful and for that reason received favor all of her life. Additionally, she was the younger sibling and the younger child is typically catered to a little more than the older child. The Bible states that Jacob loved Rachel beyond words. Think about it, he must have truly loved her because he worked 14 years to receive her hand in marriage. That's a powerful love that undoubtedly gave her tremendous favor with Jacob when it came to choosing between her and Leah.

But now, the tables were turned. Leah was conceiving and having sons left and right. She was the one helping to carry on the family name and Rachel was left with nothing. As a result, Rachel became jealous. Leah may not have helped the situation by flaunting her sons in front of Rachel, but God was teaching Rachel about trusting in Him. Rachel blamed everyone for her barrenness. She blamed herself, her sister and her husband, but it was not until much later that she turned to God. And wouldn't you know it—when she turned to God, He remembered her and blessed her womb.

Are you ready to accept God's design instead of your desire? In the days of the Bible, barrenness was seen as God's favor not being upon you. However, that wasn't it at all. God wants everyone to be fruitful and multiply. He wants to bless us all with the fruit of our wombs. For some of you, God is changing you, changing some things in your life, changing your faith and changing your thoughts about God.

A good example is when God leaves you in a trial for awhile, maybe even for several years. It can feel like you're in an oven and the temperature inside keeps rising. The hotter the temperature, the more impurities fall off from the heat. God likes to remove some of the junk from your life, so He can begin to see Himself when He looks at you. The Bible says that all of us were created in His image. For some of us, once we examine ourselves, pray to God for help and allow Him to conform us to His image, then He will bless our womb. Others will face this trial of infertility and see it as just another obstacle they'll have to fight through, only refusing to conform to His image. As a result, the blessing of a baby gets delayed even longer. For those of us who realize that God is doing something new in our lives, God tugs at our hearts in order to change us and get our attention.

Let's take a look at some common desires that women have versus God's design for our lives.

Our Desire—Love of a child

I want someone to love. I want a little baby to hold, to take care of and cuddle, or I want someone who looks like me and my husband. A baby will love me unconditionally and accept me for who I am. A baby will not judge me or make light of my faults and/or my failures.

God's Design—Focus on the Love of God

Your first desire should always be to love the Lord, your God with all your heart and make Him first in your life. If your desire to have a baby is greater than your desire to please God, then your priorities are out of focus. Have you ever thought that maybe God wants you to lay down your wants and desires and focus solely on what He wants from you in this situation?

I know you are experiencing hurt and depression because you have not conceived a child. God wants to know if you are willing to lay all of that down in order to get what He wants to give you. Your desire must match God's plan. Maybe, God has something else for you right now. You might not understand His timing or His plan, but remember He always has His best intentions for you.

In order to love another human being, you must first love God and then yourself. God loves us with an all encompassing love called "agape love". Agape love is defined as God's unconditional love. *John 15:13 says, "Greater love has no one than this, that one lay down his life for his friends."* Perhaps, in your own family setting you have never really experienced love. However, if you are a daughter of the King, then you have experienced true love. When God gave His son, Jesus Christ for our sins, this was and is the greatest love of all. Jesus, the obedient son seeking to please His father, willingly laid down his life for the world. By just repeating the previous scripture over and over and concentrating on the words should help you feel his love.

You might say, "Yes, I am grateful for that, but I can't feel his love." My response to you is "Have you ever tried?" Can you put aside your own agenda and focus your full attention on what God did for you? Have you read the Bible and found scriptures that relate to God's love and meditated on them. If not, then maybe you should. We so often want God to bless us and give us more, but God wants to give us more of Him not things, or babies. In Him we find true joy, true peace and true love. He wants to know that you want Him, not just the things He can provide.

Our Desire—Our Maternal Instinct

It's the right time—I am financially, emotionally and physically stable. I'm the right age. My life is not complete without a child.

God's Design—Focus on His Paternal Will

So often, we're caught up in our own timing. However, we fail to consider our timing in relation to God's will. You see, God's timing is everything and it all evolves around His will for our lives. Is it God's will for us to have children? Yes, His Word says to be fruitful and multiply. But His Word does not say that you will be able to produce life on your own terms, wherever and whenever you choose. God decides when your family will expand and He decides how. But first and foremost, we have to find out His will for our lives. He may not bless you with a baby right now because He may decide that He has something else for you to do right now. Instead, He may decide to bless you next year or three years or 10 years from now. We can't question His timing because He is the Father of time. He can do with time exactly what He wishes to do.

In talking with many women enduring this struggle, I find it interesting that some don't think God is going to bless their wombs. Who told you that God wasn't going to bless you? That's not what the Bible says, in fact, in Ephesians 3:20, it states, *"Now unto Him who is able to do exceeding abundantly beyond all that we ask or think according to the power that works within us, to Him be the glory in the church and in Christ Jesus to all generations forever and ever."* God is able to bless us beyond our wildest dreams. But for some of us, our blessing involves us denying our will in exchange for His will.

This means we must be broken and that's not easy. But until you are serious about God's will, and not just your own will, you will never know what God is trying to show you. This trial could be the start of a new life for you, including renewed spiritual growth and maturity in Christ. But some of you would rather test your ovulation, take your temperature and have sex as often as possible just on the off chance that you might get lucky. I'm a living witness, you can do all of those things and more, but God will not bless you until you surrender. Through my own battle with infertility, God has shown Himself and revealed tidbits of what He has in store for me. The only stipulation is that I had to replace my will with His.

The fact is, it's an easy thing for God to make a baby. From the very words of His mouth, He created both heaven and earth. That which was void of life was spoken into being. This same God can surely take two individuals, husband and wife, and make a baby from them. It all depends on you. Will you submit to whatever God wants for your life, even if it does not involve blessing you with a baby right now? You must realize that God will not bless you in your area of want until you surrender to Him what He wants.

Our Desire—Well, Everyone Else Has A Baby

Conversation:

Liz: "Girl, when are ya'll going to have some kids? Life's not complete without kids."

You: "We've been trying, but we haven't had any luck yet."

Liz: "Girl, you better hurry up, Nikki's got two kids. Mia's got two kids and another on the way. And Carla has a little boy. If you don't have children, soon, your kids won't have anyone to play with."

Everyone else has a baby. Is this really a true statement or does it just seem like everyone has a baby? Studies show that more than 6.1 million women suffer from infertility. So it doesn't sound like everyone has a baby. How many times have you been told that it's time for you to have some kids? Aren't you tired of hearing that? So many times, we let society, family and friends dictate to us what we should be doing. How many times have we sought advice from people and found that they were completely wrong about our situation.

If God has a plan for our lives, why can't we just follow His plan? So often we feel the need to develop our own plans or allow others to develop them for us. I am guilty of this myself. I was told by others to complete school, start a successful career, get married, be married for two years, then buy a house and have two children. And heaven forbid if this was not all accomplished by the time I hit age 35. Well, that did not happen the way I had anticipated. Instead, God did not bring me my husband until He thought I was ready to have a husband. My plan was a worldly plan that I had inherited from others, but that was not God's plan. Pray for and learn to develop discernment, so you will be able to determine Godly advice from self-serving advice.

God's Design—Focus on Trusting Him

Trusting God is difficult when you believe that He is blessing everyone else except you. Trust involves having faith in God even when you don't see the blessing. Knowing that God can bless your womb, but as of yet, He has chosen not to is very hard to accept. But, we can't get caught up in our feelings. We must turn away from those feelings and focus on trusting what God has said and believing that He will bless you with your own child. When you start to question whether God hears you or whether He will bless you, focus on this scripture: Proverbs 3:5-6 *"Trust in the Lord with all your heart and do not lean on your own understanding. In all your ways acknowledge Him, and He will make your paths straight."*

Isn't it funny, the love we want from a baby is the same love that God provides for us. We want a baby to love us for who we are, when God already does. We want to hold a baby and love it tenderly, when God holds us daily and provides love to us in everything we do. We want a baby because our maternal instincts tells us it's time, when God only wants our attention so He can reveal His will to us for our lives.

But many of us watch new mothers receive the babies that they've longed for, in silence, painfully tired of waiting for our own little miracle. The reality of our desire seems so far out of reach. "When will I get to have a baby shower? When will I get to shop in the maternity section or when will I get to hold my own child?" God knows and wants to acknowledge these facts, but the focus of our faith must be on trusting Him alone.

3

Determined to be Dedicated

1 Corinthians 15:58 Be steadfast, immoveable, always abounding in the work of the Lord, knowing that your toil is not in vain in the Lord.

As Kim walks through the sliding door, she quickly grabs a basket and heads for the produce aisle. Looking down at her list, she reads: "bananas, strawberries, celery, yogurt, broccoli, Honey Nut Cheerios® and salmon." She begins to think, "If this body is going to house a baby, it's going to be the best house on the block!" Kim's doctor had always told her to eat well and take her prenatal vitamin, that's all he asked. Kim is in great spirits because she knows God is going to bless her womb, but she also realizes that she has to do her part. Throughout this process, Kim is determined to be dedicated to her goal.

Are you giving God something to work with? Make sure you are doing all you can do while you wait for Him to bless you. Make no mistake, God is all powerful and truly doesn't need your help. However, He does honor your effort. How you possess your temple is very important to God.

"Temple? What temple is she talking about?"

I'm so glad you asked. God says that the body is the temple of the Holy Spirit, and each of us is responsible for that temple. God wants you to take care of yourself, inside and out. Taking care of yourself is another way you show faith. So when God blesses your mind and your body, you will be ready to receive His blessing. Are you giving God your best? Are you giving God the best of your mind, body and soul?

At this moment, how do you feel about the fact that God has not blessed you with a baby? Are you mad at God, upset with yourself or fearful that God may never answer your prayers? Search your mind and emotions and explore exactly how you feel. Tell your Heavenly Father your innermost feelings. Remember, you're His daughter and He loves you.

After you've explored your feelings and poured out your heart to God, pray that He will take the hurt away. Know in your mind that as of yet, He has not blessed you, but He will. He cannot lie. He loves and wants the best for you. And when people ask you if you have any children or inquire as to why you don't, stand tall and say "I am waiting on God." No one can refute God. Don't hold your head down and mope about it. That shows God and others that you are defeated and you really don't believe that He will or He can bless you with a child.

From my own experiences, I don't have the best "poker-face." There were times in my own struggle with infertility that I just couldn't hide my disappointment or disguise my sadness. The mind is a powerful tool, be positive, happy and expect God to bless your womb. The word says, *"Make a joyful noise all ye nations"*. Even now as I write this book to you ladies, Satan is ever present causing me to question—Why are you writing this book? No one will read it if you do not give birth to a child. But I stand on the blood of the lamb, confident that God will bless my womb with a child. I write these words out of obedience to my Heavenly Father. Satan only knows here and now, he is not omniscient like God. God knows what will happen today, tomorrow and next week.

This book must be so powerful because I am constantly attacked every time I begin to write. You see ladies, as I write this book, my faith is strengthened and renewed. This book reminds me of God's promises for my life. Now after being so rudely interrupted by Satan, I can continue. Your mind is a powerful tool and Satan loves to use the mind for his handiwork. He uses the mind to deceive us. Remember, he is a trickster, he can cause you to think about things in a different or negative light. You must protect your mind at all times because he loves to stir you up and take you down a path of his choosing. Stay focused, remember you are a daughter of a King. If God loves and feeds the birds and lilies of the field, how much more does He love you? Have Bible verses memorized and ready to use when Satan attacks, like *Jeremiah 29:11 "I know the plans I have for you, not for calamity or poverty, but a hope and a future."*

Mirror God's word back to Him. You accomplish this by taking the promises of God and reading them back to Him using your name. For example: "God knows the plans He has for Kim, not for calamity or poverty, He has a hope and a future for Kim."

The next area you need to pay great attention to is the body. After we decided again to try to conceive, I decided I needed to lose weight. I gained weight two years after I had my first miscarriage. I slowly ate myself into a depression and gained an extra 30 pounds. When I decided to lose weight, I lost 21 pounds and was content. However, medical studies have shown that if you are too thin or too overweight, your body is not as receptive to pregnancy. This makes perfect sense because I believe God wants us to be healthy, no matter your body type.

So I lost weight and drank 48 to 64 ounces of water a day. Water is great because it flushes the impurities out of your system. I watched the number of sweets and curtailed those along with caffeine. Caffeine is also seen as a conception blocker. However, I continued to eat healthy, included lots of green vegetables and fresh fruits in my diet. I was concerned about the amount of calcium intake; so I bought yogurt and had that two to three times a week. I wanted my body so well nourished that a baby would love to be in my womb. My husband said I was creating a "baby wonderland" and that was exactly what I was doing. I began taking regular vitamins, then I switched to prenatal vitamins and then I switched back again to regular vitamins. I was told by a close friend of mine to try Geritol® tonic because it goes straight into your bloodstream. She knew a lady who tried this technique and was pregnant the next month. So I took the tonic, I figured it couldn't hurt, plus it was packed full of vitamins and nutrients. Now I have to tell you, if you take Geritol® tonic, it tastes awful, but you get used to it after awhile.

Exercise is also important, but it was my toughest battle. Begrudgingly, I went to the gym as much as I could and worked out at home. I continued to walk in the expectation of my blessing. One sign of sure faith is walking in a sea of expectation. I didn't know when He was going to bless me. I just knew that He would bless me.

4

Doubting → Disappointment → Desertion

Jeremiah 29:11—"For I know the plans that I have for you, declares the Lord, plans for welfare and not for calamity to give you a future and a hope".

Kim wakes up and gazes at the calendar, it's the first of the month. She sits up in her bed and looks with hopeful thoughts that maybe this will be the month she conceives. Climbing out of her bed, the morning news plays in the background. She begins to think about the tasks she must complete today. She makes the bed and listens to a commercial advertising an EPT pregnancy test. She watches the happy couple as they read the results of their test. It's positive! They are astounded at this wonderful news. Kim can only imagine that one day this commercial will be her reality.

She starts to daydream about that day, where she would prepare a special meal for her husband. Over dinner she attempts to remain calm as she tells her husband she is pregnant. Instead she bursts with excitement as she shares the news of their new baby. Her husband is elated, patting her belly and speaking loving words to their unborn child. Everything in her life is perfect and she finally sees the end of her struggle.

Then the alarm clock sounds, and quickly she is jolted back into reality, doubting that her dream will ever come true. She is disappointed by the start of her day, but believes that God is going to bless her with a baby. The question is, "When?" She showers, eats breakfast, kisses her husband goodbye and is off to another day at work. Driving to work, she stops at a light and peers into a car next to her. There is a young mother yelling for her kids to sit down in the backseat. Instantly, she passes judgment against the mother, "When I'm a mother, I will never yell at my children. How could any mother yell at her kids when it takes so much to conceive them?" Kim dreams of the day when she will lavish her child with hugs and kisses and lots of words of encouragement. She knows that when God blesses her, she's going to be a good mommy. Arriving at work, she gets out of the car, straightens her suit, and grabs her purse and attaché case. She makes a promise not to think about babies for the rest of the day.

As she walks into the office, she is greeted by coworkers who are busy hanging balloons and streamers all over the office. "What's going on?" she asks. Her coworker reminds her, "It's Megan's baby shower, don't you remember? We talked about it yesterday and you were going to get here early to help decorate." Kim completely forgot about the baby shower and her promise to help decorate. Immediately, she apologizes, but feels ashamed, embarrassed and now depressed. She wanted to help decorate, but as tears quickly filled her eyes, she knew she couldn't. Shutting the door behind her, she goes into her office and sobs into her hands, "God, why have you deserted me?"

Doubting

What does doubting mean? Doubting means to be uncertain about an issue, refuse to believe or to call something into question. In this life, doubting is easy to do; we allow doubt to enter into every aspect of our lives. We doubt that we will receive a promotion; we doubt that we will be healed. We doubt the people in our lives, their motives and/or feelings toward us. We doubt whether God will answer our prayers and deliver our children to us. Most of us, even Christians, live our lives in a state of doubt. One important aspect about doubting that we need to remember is that it can take us to places we never imagined we would travel. Once thoughts are developed, they tend to grow into doubts and these doubts play over and over in our mind. These doubts turn into scenarios and cause our mind to take part in all types of unproductive activity—always focusing on the negative possibilities or consequences that might or might not come to pass.

Recognizing the Voice of Doubt

Have we ever thought about why these thoughts don't play positive scenarios for our lives? Think about this, out of all the thoughts we've had over the years, for the most part, why is it that most of them have negative consequences? Is there a reason for this?

Part II discusses the Daddy and daughter relationship, where we will analyze and understand our position in Christ. A lot of times, doubt shows up because we have an improper view of ourselves and of God. We create the voice of doubt because we fail to understand who God is and how His deity defines who we are. Accountability is the key if we are to ever recognize the voice of doubt. For years, many of us have allowed thoughts, doubts and scenarios into our minds that do not line up with the word of God. Doubting is human nature and everyone does it, but when doubt enters we must remind ourselves of what God says about our thoughts.

The Bible says in *2 Cor. 10:5*, "*...we are taking every thought captive to the obedience of Christ.*" This means we must guard our heart and mind against thoughts that are not of God. We must stay on guard for doubting thoughts and stop them before they take root in our lives. Now some of you are probably saying that not all doubt is all bad. For example, you believe that God sent doubt into your mind while you were dating. You started doubting whether you should continue to date a guy because you saw that he did not have your best interest at heart. Now some may believe that this doubt was from God. This is not doubt, but divine revelation. Divine revelation is when God reveals hidden truths about people, things or situations in order for us make correct and wise decisions for our lives. So, closely examine whether a thought it is doubt or revelation? If some of you are still unsure, the best way to examine doubt is to line it up with the word of God.

If you are thinking, "I'll never have a baby, nothing good ever happens to me." Does that statement line up with God's word? No, God's word says every good and perfect gift comes from above, which means good things do happen to you. Or you might say, "The doctors said my womb will not be able to sustain a baby and I will never have a child." Does that line up with God's word? No, see *Genesis 20:17-18*, "*Abraham prayed to God and God healed Abimelech and his wife and his maids, so that they bore children. For the Lord had closed fast all of the wombs of the household of Abimelech because of Sarah, Abraham's wife."* Now you can read this story yourself, but the main point is: if God closed their wombs and then opened their wombs, what can He do with ours? Therefore, God is no respecter of person. What He has done for others, He will do the same for you.

Consequences for Failure to Recognize the Voice of Doubt

When we refuse to recognize that in many instances we create the voice of doubt and allow negative possibilities to bury themselves in our minds and souls, then we bring forth an unfruitful harvest. The consequences of doubting are dangerous for two reasons: 1) God is not glorified or pleased with our doubting and 2) doubting provides fertile ground for Satan to plant his lies and watch them grow. Let's examine how God feels about doubt in the Bible, *Romans 14:23 says, "But he who doubts is condemned if he eats, because his eating is not from faith; and whatever is not from faith is sin."* Examine our doubting closely because God says it is sinful. I was a huge doubter and this was an area of my walk with Christ that I worked on constantly. Since we know that God and Satan like the opposite things in life, who do we think wants us to doubt more than anyone? That's right, Satan. So if we doubt, then we are providing Satan with ground to cultivate and we should evict him out.

Please don't misunderstand me. I know what it feels like to want a baby so badly and feel like it's never going to happen. However, realizing that doubting is a deliberate invitation for Satan to enter into the mind, we should think twice about what we hold in our thoughts. I don't think any of us wants to give Satan control of our mind, thus, allowing him to control us.

Focusing only on what we see

There are many reasons people doubt, but I'm going to talk about three. The first reason many people doubt is because they only allow themselves to focus on what they see. For most of us, we will wait for awhile, but if we don't see an answer or solution to our problem by a certain time, then we fall head first into a doubting stance. The reason this happens is because if we don't see it, then we don't believe it will happen. If you are a Christian, this concept is in direct conflict with the very definition of faith.

"Now faith is the substance of things hoped for, but the evidence of things not seen" (Hebrews 11:1). Right now, we are hoping and praying for a baby. How-

ever, we don't see a baby. Because we don't see a baby, we are becoming fearful that we may never have one. But look at what the rest of the scripture says, "*...for by it the men of old gained approval.*" In other words, God was pleased with them and approved of them because of their faith. How many times have we said jokingly, "I'll believe it when I see it." That is, in essence, what most of us believe. We are into a "show me" mentality instead of a faith mentality.

Let me give you an example: We take our car to a mechanic because the car is not functioning properly. If the mechanic tells us the compressor on our car is out, we believe him. He might go as far as to take us out to our car and have us look under the hood and show us the problem. And if we are like most women, we have no idea at what we are looking, but we believe in him because he is an expert and he knows more about our car then we do. Imagine if we believed God as easy as we believe that mechanic. If we did believe God, He would not have any trouble molding and shaping us and we would not have any trouble trusting what God told us. We have more faith in a mechanic working on our cars than a God working on our lives.

Or, maybe I should use an example closer to home. We visit our doctor and he tells us that because of our medical history, it will be hard to conceive or we may never conceive a child. We put so much stock in what that doctor is telling us because he graduated from medical school and has degrees mounted to his wall; we figure he must know what he is talking about. But we forget who supplied the knowledge to even create the medical school. We forget the doctor received knowledge only because God's grace provided him the ability to do so. Instead, we stake our last claim on what the doctor said and forget about the physician who molded us from miry clay and blew breath into our body. We forget completely about Him.

There are so many things that we cannot see, but we rely and stake our claim on them. We can't see the wind blow, but we know it does because we can feel it. I cannot see my husband's heart beating, but I know it is because he is alive and well. We must get away from this notion that I must see it mentality. We might not have enough faith to see ourselves pregnant, but we must have enough faith to know that God's power can cause us to be pregnant. Don't you know that God is able to call into being that which does not exist (Romans 4:17). God spoke and this world came into existence. What can He speak into our bodies?

Can you imagine if God allowed us to live before He created the world? We would probably walk around saying, "there's nothing you can do with this; its' always been dark and void. Nope, that's just the way it is here."

Imagine a conversation with God:

God—"I am going to create heaven and earth and populate it with animals, people, vegetation and water. It's going to be a wonderful creation."

Your response—"Are you kidding me? There is no way you can turn this around. You got nothing to work with."

God—Oh, I don't need anything to work with, I will just speak what I want to see into existence and it will happen. It will be good."

Your response—"Ok, we'll see, but don't be upset if I tell you I told you so".

The whole idea of "seeing is believing" is nonsense. We have to begin seeing things in our mind. God envisioned His creation in His mind and followed through with His plan.

Let me make my point clear. We are not God, but we should have faith in God. Just because we cannot physically see the victory does not mean we won't have the victory. Do you realize that we have more faith in the natural world than we do in the spiritual world? This is a complete contradiction. The spiritual world caused the natural world to come into being. We have to start seeing ourselves victorious in everything we do. Begin by seeing your blessing in the spirit even before it manifest in the natural. Keep in mind, just because you cannot see your answer doesn't mean it's not in the works.

When you hear yourself saying "How is it that I can be successful in everything I touch in life, except this area?" Or, "How come I can't do anything right? I seem to fail at everything." Remember to focus on the spirit world, not only on what you see. A good spiritual practice is to take God's scripture, particularly ones pertaining to children and read these back to Christ. By performing this exercise, it will increase your faith in God and in His spirit world. It doesn't matter how many times you have prayed, remove doubt from your mind. Perhaps your faith was like mine, you believe in God and the power of God, but maybe not in this area. Don't let these thoughts or emotions cause you to focus solely on the natural, take your thoughts a little higher and focus on the spirit realm and what you can't see.

I know the feeling of not having a baby and not knowing when you will have a baby is indescribable. The pain in our hearts cannot be told with words, only with tears. For us, living in doubt and disappointment is a part of our daily lives. Even though I doubted that God would bless my womb, God's voice kept reassuring me that I would have a baby soon. Although, I had this assurance, I still doubted because I did not see it. I invite you to listen to what God is saying to you. Don't doubt Him, take Him at his word. Be sure that what you are hearing is from God and not you. Sometimes we want to hear from God so much that we believe we heard him when, in fact, we really heard ourselves. Again, remember to take every thought captive and line it up with what God's word says.

We question whether we heard the voice of God

The second reason we doubt is because we are not sure that we heard the voice of the Lord. Have you ever felt that you knew God spoke to you? But later found out or believed that you did not hear God correctly. I mean you were positive that you heard from God, and then suddenly, you were skeptical about what you thought you heard. Let me give you an example of what I mean. Below is an example of a conversation that I continued to have with myself during my season of infertility.

It was spring 2001 and I had been trying to get pregnant for about three years. My cycles varied, some 28 days, some 22 days. Sometimes I ovulated and some I did not. It seemed as if the journey of pregnancy was never going to happen for me. I believed with all my heart that God was going to bless my womb with a baby, but now I was starting to question what I heard from God. Did I hear Him wrong? Or, maybe I didn't hear Him at all. Maybe it was really me talking instead of God. I know that He told me I was going to conceive and get pregnant, but maybe I didn't know anything. Maybe it wasn't God that I heard at all. Is it possible that I was confused or that I heard myself telling me this instead of God?

At this point, I couldn't be sure of anything. I had to be honest with myself, I heard God wrong. I talked to my husband and he too thought maybe we heard God wrong. Maybe God wanted us to adopt? So because we wanted a baby so badly and we wanted to honor God, we contacted the adoption agency and started down the road to adoption.

You know, it's so hard when you don't know what God wants you to do. You feel like He is placing you on one road; and then later you feel like He is placing you on another. Without answers from heaven, all we could do was wait. I felt like I was an airplane in the sky, circling, waiting to land, but no one was listening on the radio to give me clearance to land. We were in a holding pattern, wondering if God would open or close the door to adoption or allow me to become pregnant. Those were the questions we were asking ourselves and God. All we seemed to hear from heaven was silence.

After several months of the charting of cycles, again doubt slowly crept its way into our minds. We were at a crossroads, not sure whether to adopt or try to stay the course to get pregnant. We had been told that because of the endometriosis, I could become sterile. I had started believing that it had affected my fertility. Fear crept in and stayed. Because we did not understand what God was doing in our lives, we began to look inwardly at ourselves for reasons why this was happening to us. Fear caused us to wonder if we were being punished.

My husband really began to search his soul for answers. In the past, he had agreed to an abortion in a previous relationship and thought that maybe God was punishing him now because he did not speak up. He knew the abortion was wrong and felt in his heart that he should not have allowed it. Instead, he saw it as an easy way out and allowed himself to be talked into doing nothing. Even though, he has repented from this act, it has haunted him ever since. I looked at myself and could not determine why I was being punished. I was not perfect, but I was not a bad person either. I was so confused and upset because I thought I heard God's voice. Then I believed I didn't, I only heard my voice. Doubt was ever present in my heart and on my face.

The Bible says in *James 1:6-8*, *"But he must ask in faith without any doubting, for the one who doubts is the like the surf of the sea, driven and tossed by the wind. For that man ought not to expect that he will receive anything from the Lord, being a double-minded man, unstable in all his ways."*

After remembering this verse, I felt worse, we were not being punished. I doubted God, when I should have been exercising my faith. Thank God, His mercy steps in. Even when we have been told not to doubt and we do it anyway, God provides His mercy and grace to help us get through any trial. My husband and I talked about this and decided that we were going to have faith in God that whatever His will was for us, we would trust Him. We believed that his voice told us to adopt and our faith grew stronger. We were convinced that God wanted us to adopt and realized that there were so many children out there that needed a good, nurturing and safe home.

In August 2001, we contacted an adoption agency and began the process of adoption. We completed the application, prepared our profile for the birth mother, paid a $2500 deposit and completed our home visit interviews. We had the peace of God upon our lives, everything was in balance. We knew God's direction for our lives and we were content with what His will was for us. He wanted us to adopt and give a child a great life and we were all for that. We praised God even more so because He chose us to help with His plan. We were determined to make sure that the child would be loved and adored and that he would know his birth mother made a loving choice as well.

We wanted a boy and began purchasing items generic in color for our new addition. We even painted the baby's room baby blue and placed clouds at the top of the walls, so when he looked up he could see God's beauty and peace. We had it all planned and had even chosen a name for our new baby boy in hopes that he would arrive to us by Christmas Day. I purchased a few books in order to teach him the basics ABC's and 123's. We received questions about why we were adopting and we proudly stated that this was God's will for us and that we were glad to follow His plan.

But something was happening to me physically, I couldn't explain it, but all was not well. By October 2001, I was becoming increasingly more concerned about my cycles. For a couple of months, I was having a cycle every 18 days. I was still checking my ovulation but with the shortness of my cycles, I was not ovulating which I knew was a problem.

I went to the doctor for an exam and furnished him with the information regarding the number of days in my cycles along with the months I ovulated and the months I did not. He scheduled me for surgery in November 2001. My doctor advised me that because of his area of practice, he was quite familiar with the types of conditions I was experiencing. He was confident that he would have no problem solving my issue.

My husband and I became confused once again. I remembered what God told me before, about blessing my womb. The Bible says in, *Romans 4:20-21,* *"Yet with respect to the promise of God, he did not waiver in unbelief but grew strong in faith, giving glory to God and being fully assured that what God had promised He was able also to perform."* I had allowed myself to question what I heard and God was reminding me of His promise again.

Fear

The third reason we doubt is because of fear. Doubting is safe because we can always say "Oh, I never believed it would happen anyway." Did you know that doubt leads to fear and fear leads to unbelief? You might say that's a stretch, but trust me my friend, it's not. One doubt can change our whole perspective of a situation. When doubt festers, it gives birth to fear, and fear gives birth to unbelief. Once we lack belief in our situation, it becomes hopeless and pretty soon we're hopeless, too. Fear is anxiety caused by a real or possible danger or pain or apprehension. I know that many are heartbroken and your feelings are hurt. I have been where you are, but I have also overcome and you can too.

What do we fear? For some of us, we have allowed fear to take over our minds because we have miscarried or given birth to a stillborn baby. Let's talk about fear and how fear encases itself around our being, particularly in a miscarriage. We find out we're pregnant and we're so excited. We even share our news with others and they are excited for us. Then our body decides to reject the fetus and we miscarry. As we watch this physical scene of blood and tissue flowing from our bodies, we're devastated and never want to relive it again. The physical part of a miscarriage is painful and not pleasant to see, but it's nothing compared to the emotional side of a miscarriage.

It's the emotional side that constantly plagues us. We see babies at the mall and wonder why our baby miscarried. We are reminded nine months later of our baby's due date if he or she had lived. For some of us, years later we can count how old our baby would have been. Miscarriages are rough. They shake our whole world and demonstrate our total lack of control. Don't get me wrong, miscarriages can be overcome with Christ. I've had two miscarriages and I was devastated by each one.

My first miscarriage occurred in February 2000 and I allowed myself to wallow in pity. I closed myself off from everyone except my husband and immediate family. While I continued to pray to God, I was actually disappointed with God. I felt as though God could have done something to save my baby, but He didn't. I spent my time wondering "why" instead of accepting God's will.

I spent two years in a secret depression. For me, life seemed to be running in slow motion. Sure, everyone saw the outer Kim, but no one knew the pain that I felt inside. I continued to smile and provide interesting conversation, but when I was alone, I knew it was all just a show. I was surprised that nobody even noticed that I was only going through the motions. With most of my acquaintances, I was there with them physically, but my mind was stuck peering through the rails of a baby bed. My thoughts were on so many different issues and all of it surrounded my failure to become a mother. At the end of that two year depression, I found myself 30 pounds heavier and disgusted with my happy facade. It was at that point that I decided to wake up. I began examining fear and faith as I contemplated my life. God began speaking to me and helping me to understand these terms.

Fearful contemplation is being indecisive about venturing forward due to an event or a situation that has caused us pain or hurt in the past. Fearful contemplation causes us to be stagnant and afraid to move in any direction. If I do this, then something bad will happen. For example, if I try to become pregnant, I might not conceive. Even worse, if I try to become pregnant, I could have another miscarriage and I can't let that happen again; so I won't even try. In essence, we're protecting ourselves from hurt.

But what if a miscarriage doesn't occur this time? What if you carry the baby full term and deliver a healthy baby? Many of you will never know because you're stuck in a fearful way of life. If I don't try to get pregnant, then I can ensure myself that I will never hurt like that again. You may be missing out on your blessings. Let's remind ourselves of what God says about fear in *Isaiah 41:10, "Do not fear, for I am with you; do not anxiously look about you, for I am your God. I will strengthen you, surely I will help you, surely I will uphold you with My righteous right hand."* God is telling us in this passage not to fear, but look to Him because He is always with us and will always help us. Instead of focusing on fearful contemplation, we should focus on **faithful contemplation**. Of course this concept relies on your level of faith. Faithful contemplation is positive reflection on God's goodness in your life. Faithful contemplation causes you to move forward by faith, regardless of the outcome, because you trust God and have faith that God has a purpose and a plan for everything. God always sustains you through whatever you go through. Step out and trust God by practicing faithful, not fearful contemplation.

Disappointment

God's word says in *Romans 5:3-5,; "And not only this, but we also exult in our tribulations, knowing that tribulation brings about perseverance, and perseverance, proven character; and proven character, hope; and hope does not disappoint, because the love of God has been poured out within our hearts through the Holy Spirit who was given to us."* We were all set to adopt and now our reality of adoption was being called into question. We had heard before that we had a clean bill of health and we should be able to conceive. However, it had not happened in the past; so it was hard for us to entertain the thought of it happening in the future. We had to question what we believed about His will for our lives. We just knew that God wanted us to adopt and now a doctor was telling us something different. We didn't know whether we should trust the word of the doctor or trust what we thought we heard from God. Eventually, we stepped out on faith—once again contacting the adoption agency. We explained that I had to have another surgery and asked if they would place us on their inactive list. They agreed and we continued to pray for answers.

Going back to the scripture above, it states that hope does not disappoint. So, why were we disappointed? We had taken our eyes off God and focused on our situation from an earthly perspective. Remember the story in Matthew where Peter asked Jesus if he could walk on the water with Him. Peter started walking on the water as he continued to focus on Jesus and moving toward Him. Suddenly, the wind came, Peter lost his focus, became frightened and began to sink (Matthew 14:28-31).

That's exactly what happened to us, we took our eyes off God and looked to man. As you can imagine, when we did this, our faith began to sink. We should have been listening and leaning on God, not on ourselves and what we saw. The above scripture also talks about exulting in our tribulations, but we did not do that either. Instead, we allowed our trial to speak to us when we should have been speaking God's word back to the trial. Although we truly wanted a baby from our womb, it seemed possible; however, our lack of faith only allowed us to believe that God could only bless us through adoption.

I wrote God a letter regarding my confusion, my doubt and my faith:

11/23/01

Dear God,

I began this journey by praising You God for Your awesome mercy and wisdom. You have not allowed us to conceive and give birth to a child. We believed that you wanted us to adopt, so we started that process and then you threw us a curve ball (I got sick). My surgery is scheduled for 11/28/01 at 11:00 a.m. You have given us a doctor who is competent and confident. We were on one road and now you have placed us on another.

We are a bit confused, but understand that you have a reason for everything you do. We want to follow your lead. We are not sure what lies ahead, but we are sure of whom You are and that only You know what lies ahead. I have purchased some books on faith to help me prepare my mindset for what you have in store for us. Father, cleanse me and grant me wisdom as I read, study and memorize biblical principles that You have laid out for me in these books and in Your Holy Word, the Bible.

Yours in Faith,

Kim

P.S. Help my unbelief!!!

Remembering the beginning of this chapter, I talked about doubt leading to fear and fear leading to unbelief. Look at my P.S. at the end of my letter, "Help my unbelief." That's what I am talking about; my doubt took me all the way to a lack of faith in God. I actually asked Him to help me believe in Him.

That's why you have to be so careful with thoughts of doubt. Before you know it, you're questioning God and whether or not you truly believe what He says. Realizing my error, I turned my focus away from doubt and made a conscious decision to believe God and have faith. I read *Mark 11:23-24* over and over. It states, *"Truly I say to you, whoever says to this mountain, Be taken up and cast into the sea and does not doubt in his heart but believes that what he says is going to happen, it will be granted to him. Therefore I say to you, all things for which you pray and ask, believe that you have received them, and they will be granted to you."*

I began to think that maybe this time God was truly going to bless my womb. After all, my doctor was so confident in his abilities. I had this feeling once before regarding conception, but I didn't want to dwell on it. My hope became renewed in the possibility that God was going to give me a baby from my own womb. As I prayed and meditated, a thought came to me regarding Abraham in the Bible. Abraham was asked by God to sacrifice his son—taking him up a mountain and placing him on an alter the way they sacrifice animals. Abraham was told to raise the knife and kill his son. God asked Abraham to sacrifice his only son, the son that Abraham thought he would never have because of his age and because of Sarah's barrenness.

Through this vision, God showed me that He was waiting on me to sacrifice my womb for Him. He wanted to see if I could sacrifice having a child from my womb and be happy adopting. He was testing my faith to determine if I loved Him enough to still praise Him and truly be content in my circumstances without a child from my own womb. Obviously, God already knew the answer. This exercise of faith was for my benefit. He was proving my level of faith and testing me to see if I could be at peace with His decision. Could I sacrifice my own desires for His perfect will and still praise Him? God allowed me to have the wisdom and grace to demonstrate my will to praise Him. I was reminded of Paul in *Philippians 4:11, "…I have learned to be content in whatever circumstances I am."* Ironically, I experienced more peace during this time period than I had in years. I was convinced that God still wanted us to adopt, but He did not want us to rule out His power to allow us to conceive.

November rolled around and I was scheduled for surgery. This was the fourth surgery in less than two years. Needless to say, surgeries were not scary anymore. I was quite familiar with the anesthesiologist and the doctors. This particular doctor performed my DNC in 2000 after my first miscarriage. He exuded confidence. In fact, he was almost over confident. So much so that I began to piggyback on his confidence, even though I knew that it had to be God to bless my womb and not the abilities of the doctor. The surgery went well. The doctor gave me a clean bill of health and we planned to start trying again after two more cycles.

I started the New Year by writing another letter to God.

1/1/02

Dear Father,

Our surgery is complete and successful. My ovaries were pulled down from the endometriosis. As a result of them being pulled down, they were not functioning as they should. The doctor sutured my ovaries up and placed them back where they were supposed to be. He told us that because this was a highly unusual procedure that I was at a higher risk for a tubule pregnancy. But he believed that I could get pregnant in about six months, we would just have to be watchful of the possibility of a tubule pregnancy.

So, we are at Stage 1 again. I had my cycle 12/19/01, Steven and I are trying to conceive. We are timing my ovulation and preparing for your blessing of a beautiful healthy child. Thank you Lord for a successful surgery!! We are confessing our faith and believing that you are going to answer our prayers. Thank you in advance for our baby or babies.

Love Always,

Your Daughter

Kim

Desertion

In 2002, things were going fine. I was ovulating, Steven and I were timing our love making, but nothing seemed to be happening. Then I received another visit from Satan. I don't mean he stopped by my house for a chat. I mean, he entered my mind and stayed for awhile. He began to make me question and doubt God again; but this time, he came with a vengeance. Little by little, every day I began thinking, "When am I going to have a baby?" "Did I read God wrong, again?" Earlier, we had contacted the adoption agency to start adoption, then we stopped the adoption; now do we contact them again? These thoughts and others continually crept into my mind and rang in my head day and night:

Dear God,

"I feel like I am doing everything I am supposed to do. I am testing my ovulation; we are making love and praying to You for our miracle. But Father where are You? Have You deserted me? I don't feel You are with me at all. I feel alone and deserted. Do You even hear me or my prayers? I have prayed and prayed. I have tithed and tithed. I have had faith on top of faith and still <u>nothing.</u> What does all of this mean? Will I ever have children from my womb? Why are You making me wait? Is there something I need to learn? If so what is it? I want to learn whatever it is, so I can get this waiting over with and move on. God, are You real? If You were You would have answered me by now.

Do You even love me anymore? Do you care?"

Kim

I was teetering on anger with God because I was so tired of the waiting game and not knowing what was going on with my life. I needed answers and I needed them now. I had four surgeries in two years and still nothing. I was upset, but I could do nothing except continue to wait on God. I felt awful. Even more, I never picked-up the Bible to reassure myself of God's blessings. Satan had me right where he wanted me, frustrated and disgusted.

How many times have you felt alone? How many times have you felt that you were the only one going through this trial? Thank God, I had been a Christian attending a strong, faith-based church. I heard the word of God weekly. I was quickly reminded to pray and read the Word of God. Can you believe that I questioned whether God was even real? After all God had done for me, I was still questioning whether He was real.

I went back to God, asked for forgiveness, read His Word and prayed. *Hebrews 13:5-6 states, "I will never desert you, nor will I ever forsake you, so that we confidently say, The Lord is my Helper, I will not be afraid. What will man do to me?"*

Just as I was starting to renew my faith again, Mother's Day was here. My monthly cycle was a little late, of course I immediately believed that I was pregnant even though I took a pregnancy test and it was negative. I thought to myself "it's early and maybe the test hadn't picked up the pregnancy hormone yet". Anyway, we prepared to go to church. Oh how I dreaded this holiday. All the mothers of the church got to stand up and receive applause for all their valiant efforts in raising their children. I was happy for them, but sad for me. I wanted to stand up with the rest of the mothers and have my husband look at me, admiring and appreciating all I do to help raise well-balanced children. That was not the case for me; I had to remain seated year after year. But maybe this year was different, maybe my suspicions about my late cycle would be confirmed soon.

Mothers all over the sanctuary received corsages or roses as I sat with nothing in my hand. There was no corsage, no rose and no baby. There was nothing to show that I had even tried to become a mother. I even thought about boycotting this day, but I knew my husband would never go for it. I remember thinking one year, "I had a miscarriage, does that count? Can I at least stand up and be acknowledged for that." I was happy to honor mothers, but I just couldn't get past the hurt of not being a mother myself. As you might know, at the Mother's Day dinner with our families, my cycle started.

Repeatedly, I had to remind myself of *Hebrews 13: 5-6* because I was constantly allowing normal aspects of life like Mother's Day to continue to get me down. Hebrews 13 confirmed that God had not left me nor forsaken me. God had not moved away from me, but I had moved away from Him.

It's important for us to stay in prayer and in the Word of God. Satan looks for opportunities to take us off the course God has intended for each of us. We must remember that God promises to be our helper and our friend and we should not be afraid. Instead of listening to our destructive thoughts, we need to ask God for help and allow these thoughts to dissipate.

5

Decisions

Psalms 119:133—Establish my footsteps in Your word,
And do not let any iniquity have dominion over me.

We all have met and know indecisive people who go through life and are never able to make a decision. These people usually second guess their decisions and wind up changing their minds, continuously resulting in unnecessary consequences for themselves and those around them. The Bible calls these people *double-minded unstable in all their ways (James 1:8)*. Well, there is nothing double-minded or indecisive about God, He makes decisions and He stands by those decisions. You might say, all of this is good information, but how do I make the right decisions? Before you make a decision, you need to consult God and hear what He says about the facts and allow Him to direct you to the right decision and then you need to obey the decision.

In the next session, Daddy and Daughter, we will discuss how you hear from God and I will give you examples of the ways I hear from God. You have to be able to hear from God about your situation. If you say, I have never heard from God, then you should examine your relationship with Him? In God's Word, He says in *John 10:3, "The sheep hear His voice and He calls His own sheep by name and leads them out."* God knows us by name, He created us and the verse says that He leads us; we are being led by His voice, but you must hear His voice. But for most of us, this is not the case; we have heard from God, but we do not like the answer He has given us. What do you do when God's plan for your life is different than your plan for your life? Here you are, you want to have a child and have done everything within your power

41

to make this your reality. You have developed a relationship with Christ and you are completely devoted to Him. You pray and pray and still nothing. You are at a point where you are beginning to wonder if you are destined to have children. Heaven is silent; yet, you are still waiting. After awhile frustration sets in and you don't know which way to turn. Let's face it, not only are you not hearing from God, you can no longer feel God's presence in your life. You feel alone and you believe that no one can relate to your hurt, not even Jesus. When you feel yourself dwindling spiritually, that's when you must encourage yourself in the Lord. Don't allow yourself to spiral downward. The word says in *Isaiah 41:10*, *"Do not fear for I am with you; do not anxiously look about you, for I am your God. I will strengthen you, surely I will help you, surely I will uphold you with My righteous right hand"*.

Every situation that occurs in your life is predestined and ordained just for you. The great thing about God is He already knows the decisions you will make. If you are unsure of what God is saying, don't make a hasty decision on your own, instead pray and tell God that you are confused and ask for God to give you clarity on the issue. When you decide to make decisions on your own, you demonstrate a lack of faith as well as wisdom which usually leads you on a path of despair and disappointment. It is better to allow God to lead and direct you to the right decision, so that you have a positive outcome.

Why am I barren? Activate your faith—you might be saying I have activated my faith, I am a Christian and I pray everyday for a baby and God does not answer. My response to you is there maybe a couple of reasons as to why God is not answering your prayers. One may be that God is shaping your character in order to move you to His next level.

The second possible reason for your barrenness may be timing. God does everything in His own timing. Maybe God has not blessed your womb because in this season His timing dictates that you adopt. You see, God may have a holistically different approach for you than He does for someone else. It's not that He won't bless your womb; He might not think it's time because He has a child that He has birthed, earmarked for you to take care of. You don't want what God does not have for you. Get in alignment with His word and with Him. But maybe some of you have heard from God and He has already answered you, but you refuse to acknowledge Him or listen to His answer.

The Bible states that we should be fruitful and multiply and fill the earth; we have interpreted that to mean have babies, but is that all there is to that phrase or could God have two different meanings for the phrase? Could He mean have children and allow them to multiply the earth? And raise children to have fruitful lives so that they are multiplied to others by God's teaching? In this season, God may have an alternative plan for your fruitfulness. Suppose God's plan for you at this moment is adoption? Maybe God's plan for you involves giving birth from your heart? I know what you are saying, but the Bible says that I should be fruitful and multiply, but what if God wants you to adopt a child and fill that child's life; is that not considered being fruitful and multiplying? The Bible says in *Matthew 7:17-20, "So every good tree bears good fruit, but the bad tree bears bad fruit. A good tree cannot produce bad fruit, nor can a bad tree produce good fruit. Every tree that does not bear good fruit is cut down and thrown into the fire. So then you will know them by their fruits."* Suppose God wants you to adopt a child and produce good fruit; suppose He knows that if you don't adopt that child, that the child will eventually produce bad fruit? Let's just say, you have a good relationship with Christ and He has placed adoption in your heart, but you want to have your own baby from your own womb. What are you doing with that information? Are you ignoring it? Are you trying to conceive in spite of what God has told you? Could it be that you are not conceiving because He has another plan for you? Maybe God's plan is for you to adopt and then bless you with a baby from your womb? God has a plan and a purpose for everyone, but it is His plan, not ours. Don't get me wrong, God's Word says to be fruitful and multiply and I believe that God has the power and ability to cause every woman to conceive and give birth to a child, but what if God wants that for you and more. What if He is requiring you to sow a seed by adopting a child who otherwise would not have a good home? The Bible says in *Acts 10:34 that God is no respecter of persons, what He does for one, He will do the same for the other.* The above scripture indicates that it is not because He loves some more than others, He loves us all the same and He, therefore, treats us according to our needs. I know you are thinking to yourself, so why do some women die barren? I don't know the answer to this question; all I know is that when you follow God's plan for your life, it will be filled with blessings. Is it possible that God has a different plan for those women and a different plan for some children who are left without parents? Could it be that He wants them to adopt and raise children that have been orphaned, thrown away by their parents, and/or physically and emotionally abused? Could it be that He knows these mothers will take special care of them by loving and caring for them as their own? Perhaps, these mothers will be there to reassure them that they are mighty conquerors because of their relationship with Christ and to explain that all Christians have been adopted into Jesus Christ's family? And these children will have more growth potential and opportunity because of the environment that their mother and father have provided for them. I think it is an honor for God to look down and say I want her to be his/her mother because she has some qualities and characteristics that this child needs. And vice/versa, this child has some characteristics that this mother needs. To be chosen by God for this mission blesses Jesus because the Bible says whatever you do to the least of these little children, you do it unto me. By you blessing a child with a safe and secure loving home full of laughter and praise for their accomplishments, you are doing this act unto the Father. You could have ignored that voice in your heart, telling you to adopt, but you heeded the call and now you have a testimony of truly being a joyful mother; look at the rewards you will reap. Consider that it's really not about you, what if it's all about the child, but God allows you to get blessed in the process by loving that child. You never know who you could be raising; that child might be the next Billy Graham or T. D. Jakes.

Adoption for many is a difficult issue when you are trying to conceive, but instead of saying I want someone to look like me, look at it from God's perspective and how pleased He will be with your obedience. I am reminded of a story in the Bible involving Pharaoh's daughter in Exodus, Chapter 2 where Pharaoh called for all Hebrew sons to be killed at birth and all daughters to be saved. Moses' mother hid her child for three months and when she could not hide him any longer, she placed him in a basket and sent him floating down the Nile River near Pharaoh's home. And as the story goes, Pharaoh's daughter saw the basket and sent a maid to get it and there she found a beautiful baby boy nestled with a Hebrew blanket. She fell in love with him and called him her son. She loved, took care of him and educated him just as if she had given birth to him. He blessed her soul and she blessed his. What a joyful mother she must have been.

Activate Your Faith—Positively or Negatively

You can activate your faith in a positive way or a negative way, but however you choose to activate your faith in a positive way or a negative way, God responds to that choice. When you say, I will never have children, God responds Okay. We talked in previous chapters that faith is the key to God and it operates positively or negatively. Someone might say, "But it's impossible for me to get pregnant because I had to have a hysterectomy in order to save my life." All I can say is Sarah was 90 plus years old when she got pregnant. For all intents and purposes, her womb could be considered dead after all this time, but God, (notice I said but God). God can cause those things that are nonexistent to be existent, just look at the earth. In *Genesis 1:2-3, it states, "The earth was formless and void and darkness was over the surface of the deep...Then God said, Let there be light and there was light."* God spoke this earth into existence. So, if He can speak heaven and earth into existence and all its' inhabitants, don't you think He can also speak life to your belly and life come forth? We know what God has done for others, He will do the same for you. Activate your faith, believe in the power of God. Know that He has good things in store for you; know that He wants to bless you. *"Ask whatever you will in my name and it shall be granted to you".* If you are not pregnant, ask God to reveal the reason, ask Him to show you what needs to change in you and ask him about His timing and what His plans are for you. Activate your faith. God says you can speak to this mountain and it shall be moved and cast in the sea. Search your heart, soul and mind and find out what needs to be cast in the sea. God is a mighty God who created heaven and earth and all that exists in it. If He can do that He can do anything including cause your belly to bulge with a baby. Don't give up, give in to God. Search Him and search you for the answer. I tell you, He is a faithful God who delivers. Activate your faith. God is a jealous God; therefore if you are putting others or things in front of God, stop and put God first.

The third possible reason for your barrenness may be to give you a testimony. Most times, we go through struggles to help someone else. See, while you are in the struggle, you can relate to it because you have lived it. In other words, you not only sympathize, but you empathize because you know what it is like not to be able to conceive and want to more than life. You understand the feeling to constantly struggle to attend each and every baby shower, but you have to show up and try to be happy for the mother-to-be when inside, the whole scenario is eating you alive because you wish it were your baby shower.

Oh, I know what it feels like to hear children call their mothers' mommy and you feel like no one will ever call you that and give you a hug. I know because I have been there. But you see God allows us to go through struggles so we will remember who is on the throne. If everything were rosy in your life, if you never had a problem, why would you need God? You would think everything is fine, why do I need God? Sometimes, God has to get our attention with a trial, but the beautiful thing is that it is always for our good. My struggle of trying to get pregnant was hard, but look at the testimony and the blessing that came from that struggle. Now, my job is to help you cross the bridge of faith into your destiny.

6

The Deceiver

Revelation 12:9 "....Satan who deceives the whole world..."

Kim decides to go to the gym to workout. Everyone says exercising is good for you because it reduces stress and gives you more energy. Today, I need both. I arrive at the gym and step on the treadmill. I program the treadmill at my usual pace, but I forgot my headphones. Oh well, I'll just settle for watching TV. Two ladies step on treadmills next to mine; it's obvious they are friends. I was trying not to listen to their conversation, but it was loud enough for me to hear. One of the ladies started singing to the other lady, "I'm every woman...it's all in me. Everything you want done baby...I do it naturally." She talks of her husband and their two wonderful kids. It sounds like she has every woman's dream. As I listen to her, I think, "She does have it all and I have nothing."

I try to get this thought out of my mind. I start thinking about what makes me different from her. Maybe I don't have everything that she has because I'm being punished for something in my past. As I ponder this thought and allow my mind to drift, I continue to exercise. Why am I thinking this way, I can save myself a lot of heartache by just focusing on my career and forgetting about having a family. Maybe it's not for everybody. Besides, I've already had two miscarriages, what's the point of going for three.

Who is the deceiver? Many may think anyone can be a deceiver and this is a correct assumption. However, there is only one deceiver that presides over all deceivers and all deception. His name is Satan, formerly named Lucifer or some just call him the devil. *The Bible states in Genesis 3:15, "And I will put enmity between you (Satan) and the woman, and between your seed and her seed."* As you can see, virtually from the beginning of time, women have been in a fight against Satan for a very long time. Satan hates women because they have the capability to birth men and women who will serve Christ. As you might imagine, Satan doesn't want any more Christians because this makes his job harder.

Television and other forms of media portray Satan as a character who is painted red, dressed in a red suit with a pitchfork in his hands and smoke coming from his ears. But this is not who Satan is at all. He is a warrior for evil and he is real. Let me tell you a little bit about this enemy. Before there was a hell, Lucifer (Satan) was one of God's most beautiful angels. He was endowed with many powers. As a result of his great beauty and power, Lucifer began to think that he was better than God (*Isaiah 14:19*). His pride got the best of him and he convinced one third of the angels to follow him. When they did, they were cast out of heaven into the abyss. He had to be pretty influential in order to talk a third of the angels into leaving heaven and reigning with him.

It took me awhile to complete this book because Satan made me believe that no one would read it. I'm telling you this so you might understand how crafty and determined Satan is to see your demise. You need to know that Satan's powers are real. Don't ever think he's not working behind the scenes towards your ultimate failure because he is. He wants you to believe that your household will not be filled with beautiful children. He wants to silence your dream of tiny little feet running down the hallways. He wants you to believe that the sound of children's laughter will never be heard throughout your home. Satan gets into your mind and causes you to doubt yourself and God. His mission is to trick you into believing his lies about your destiny. However, we must counter each and every lie thrown our way with the truth of God. We have to remember that God made us and God is based upon truth. We must always believe God first, above everyone and everything else. Here are some of the lies that Satan has told me and other women whom I've talked:

Lie 1: "Having a baby is the most basic function of a woman, maybe I'm not a woman."

Lie 2: "I am never going to get pregnant because my past has been so bad. My sins are too great for God to bless me now."

Lie 3: "Maybe you're not meant to be a mother, focus on your career. Climb the corporate ladder to success and forget about a family."

Lie 4: "If by chance I get pregnant, I probably won't be able to bring the baby to term. I will probably miscarry again."

Satan's Lie #1
"Having a baby is the most basic function of a woman,
maybe I'm not a woman."

Analysis #1

Have you ever wondered why God made you a woman? When you struggle with trying to have a baby, this thought is bound to come to your mind. I know it came to mine. Since the most basic function of a woman is to bear children, it's understandable why we would question our inability to conceive and/or bring a baby to term. As I struggled with this concept, I came to the conclusion that this thought process left me feeling worthless, alone and many times envious of other women. Let's analyze these thoughts:

I. Worthless—Despite all of my efforts (i.e. prayer, timing ovulation, exercise, and eating right), still nothing. It's a feeling of worthlessness when you struggle trying to get something that you've wanted so badly, but you watch others get the gift without any effort or thought. It's the worst feeling on earth to question your womanhood. Some call us damaged goods because our internal wiring is all wrong. Maybe you think, "Am I a woman at all or did God make a mistake? Did I not get everything I was supposed to have? How can I even call myself a woman when by its very definition 'woman' means a female with the ability to give birth to a child."

Dear Diary,

My husband looks at me and has pity on me. Sometimes, I think he wishes he did not have to bear this burden with me. Maybe, he would have rather married someone who could give him the babies he always wanted. Yet, he says it doesn't matter if we have children or not, but you know he is only saying that to make me feel better. He doesn't mean it. He wants to see himself in his children. Who are we fooling? He wants a son who looks like him and who he can mold into his own image, I can't blame him. His ego is tied to who he is and who wouldn't want to see themselves through their child. I feel sorry for myself because there is nothing I can do. I am doing everything I know how. My mother says that if I pray, it will happen. I do so and still nothing. I'm questioning what value I bring to this marriage, to my husband, to myself. What is the point? Society's definition of family is not made up of a husband and a wife. A family includes a husband, wife and kids. We can never be a real family without kids. Once again I am worthless, there is no hope for me or my situation. I'll never have a family or a child.

Yours,

Not sure who or what I am.......?

Kim

II.   **Alone**—Who can I share my pain with? No one understands that my desire to have a baby with my husband is sometimes stronger than my desire for life itself. I have sunk into a pit that I cannot explain. Knowing that I may never conceive is excruciating pain. Wallowing in my pitiful situation leads me to feeling alone. It's just me and my cycle.

What can I do month after month? My cycle shows up and I see the blood with disappointed eyes. As I see the red blood, I also see rage that my period has caused me. I see it as the enemy. When it is present, I am constantly reminded that once again, I'm not pregnant. And while my cycle is here, it acts as a soldier fighting in combat against me. The pain and frustration are compounded every time I encounter it. The more I hate it, the more it pains me. That red blood is the reason for my worth-lessness. The pain comes at me with a vengeance because it knows I don't want it here. I serve notice on it, "Cycle, you are not welcome here."

III. **Envious**—I would like to say that I'm not envious of pregnant women or women with children, but I would be lying to you. I'm caught between emotions of being happy and jealous. On one hand, I rejoice with them, while on the other hand, I wish it were me. Watching my friends have babies left and right and attending one too many baby showers causes even more distress, but what can I do? Should I tell them that I can't come because it makes me sad? No, baby showers are a joyous occasion. Everyone is happy for the mother-to-be including me. I love children, but obviously my womb does not love me. If it did, I would have my own baby to hold. No, I'll just sit alone, wishing and hoping for my opportunity.

God's Truth #1
The Bible states in Philippians 4:6, "Be anxious for nothing but in everything by prayer and supplication with thanksgiving let your requests be made known to God."

Satan's Lie #2:
"I am never going to get pregnant because my past
has been so bad. My sins are too great and I've done
too much for God to bless me."

Analysis #2

Now, does this sound like something God would say to you? This whole statement is so negative. Nothing in it shows a sign of hope or deliverance or anything positive. Isn't it just like the deceiver to speak in the negative? Why do you think he is bringing up your past? Simple, his goal is to deter you from arriving at your place of destiny.

You see, if the deceiver can keep you bound in your past, then you will never experience the future. Your future is full of bountiful opportunities and blessings. Satan knows that if you ever really tap into God and allow Him to bless your life, then you will experience the abundantly joyous life God has in store for you.

In *Ephesians 4:22-23, it says to "lay aside the old self, which is being corrupted in accordance with the lusts of deceit, and that you be renewed in the spirit of your mind and put on the new self which in the likeness of God has been created in righteousness and holiness of the truth."* Don't you realize that this is not about what you want or your past, it's about what God can show you now about your character, your growth in Him, your trust in Him. Realize this is your time to grow in Christ, to stop drinking milk and get on solid food. You have a divine appointment with God and He is not going to let you miss it. Sure you can decide to forget it; I'll focus on my career or take up a hobby or work on my body and decide that kids are just not for me. But God is not into being ignored. He planted that desire in you for a reason and He will not leave it until He has fulfilled His purpose for that desire. God enrolls us in classes all of our lives. And just like when you progressed through school, if you did not complete the class with a passing grade, you were doomed to repeat the class until you passed it. Same scenario here, He will continue to teach you His principles until you get it or pass His course. There is no escaping or ignoring God. It's simply not an option. There is only one way, His way. So if you do not want to repeat the course, the best thing for you to do is pray, mediate and obey His Word.

When you truly experience God, then it's harder for Satan to agitate you. Your mind becomes solely focused on God and His will for your life. I call this a "God focused life," which means nothing that comes your way takes you away from the path of God. You are God focused when you're preoccupied daily with thoughts and ways to please God. God focused people are on alert because they know that the deceiver is going to send something their way to try to steal their joy. God focused people understand the spiritual realm. They understand that there are angels sent by God to protect us and watch over us. At the same time, there are demons sent by Satan to steal our dreams. They are sent to cause failure to be our constant companion. And if allowed, they will kill us. So, Satan has to work overtime to make sure that you never receive God's blessings for your life.

One way of doing that is to remind you of your past. The deceiver harps on all of our flaws and makes us feel so inadequate that we think that God will not bless us. He is a crafty creature and his biggest and best accomplishment is to make you doubt God. He wants you to believe that you are not worthy to even have a God because of who you are and what you have done. However, I have good news, your best line of defense against the deceiver is God. God wants you to confess your sins and any unrighteousness before Him. We must get everything out in the open. What is Satan using in your past to torment you? Did you have an affair with a married man? Did you have an abortion? Were you a stripper or a prostitute? Or have you been a gossiper and used your gossip to destroy others' lives? Are you a liar or a thief? I don't know what's in your past, but I know of someone who can erase the past and bring you into your present without fear and without condemnation. His name is Jesus Christ. Expose your sin and lay it down at His altar of grace for His cleansing. You cannot be forgiven or cleansed of your sins if you continue to hide them. Now realize, God sees all and knows all. You have not hidden anything from Him." God forgives us of our sins and cleanses us from all unrighteousness, look at what the Bible says in *Psalm 32:5, "I acknowledged my sin to You, and my iniquity I did not hide; I said "I will confess my transgressions to the Lord", and You forgave the guilt of my sin".*

The Bible further states in *1 John 1:9, "If we confess our sins, He is faithful and righteous to forgive us our sins and to cleanse us from all unrighteousness."* Now that we know why Satan brings up our past, let's look at how he does it. Satan uses our emotions to bring up our past. There are usually three very strong emotions that we need to examine in order to understand Satan's continued deception in our lives.

Embittered

The first emotion we experience is embitterment and it is defined as aggravation, irritation, annoyance or bothered. Why are we embittered? Well, usually we are aggravated because we don't want to talk about our past or be reminded of it in any way. Our goal is to forget about it and move on with our lives. In other words, we totally remove it from our thoughts. We begin our journey of forgetting about it, eventually we erase it from our memory; and then Satan brings it back up. This is both frustrating and aggravating especially when you thought it was over. Thus, we become embittered. Be careful, once the deceiver has you irritated, then he has you on his fishing line and is on his way to reeling you in.

Guilt

Embitterment leads to the second emotion Satan uses, which is guilt. Guilt is defined as a painful feeling of self reproach resulting from a belief that one has done something wrong or immoral. He uses guilt to bully us. Suddenly we think, "Maybe I am not getting pregnant because of things I did in my past."

Maybe you engaged in lesbianism. Or maybe you've held envy and jealousy in your heart toward women with children. We could go back and think of all sorts of things we have done with our lives. We could start with every lie we ever told and continually beat ourselves up with the guilt behind our actions. Or we could give all of our sins to God and ask Him to forgive us for each and every one. We must realize that God is not using our past to punish us now.

Philippians 3;13 states,... "forgetting what lies behind and reaching forward to what lies ahead, I press on toward the goal for the prize of the upward call of God in Christ Jesus." Look at this statement from the Bible. It is saying forget the past and reach for your future. A pastor once said, "Your past is the greatest teacher but your future is your greatest reacher." You cannot reach into your future if you are continually focusing on your past. Remember our discussion earlier regarding "God focused" people, you cannot be focused on God and His will if your mind is preoccupied with your past.

Imagine that your past is like an anchor on a boat. Now an anchor is a heavy object usually made of steel, but it is used to keep a boat from drifting. Think of an anchor wrapped around your neck. It is so heavy that you can barely carry it; and since it is so heavy, you drop it and let it drag the ground. Its weight is so heavy that it is pulling you down with it. That's what the deceiver wants your past to do to you. He wants it to debilitate you to the point of causing you not to function normally. He wants the weight of your past to bombard you to where your faith, your vision and your life are too heavy to continue carrying.

Do you see why he keeps bringing your past up? He wants to hurt you in the worst way and one of his ways of hurting you is to keep reminding you of your faults and past failures. But, you've got to stand tall and admit, "Yes, I did that in my past, I repented from that sin and I turned away from ever doing it again." Once you do this, you must realize that your past is not a predictor of your future. *Isaiah 61:10 says, "I will rejoice greatly in the Lord, my soul will exult in my God; for He has clothed me with garments of salvation, He has wrapped me with a robe of righteousness".* We should be rejoicing that God has saved us and wrapped us in a robe of righteousness. Because of Jesus Christ's sacrifice and our acceptance of Him as our Lord and Savior, we wear a robe of righteousness. This is not because of who we are, but because of who He is.

With this information, the deceiver should never be allowed to annoy us with our past. Every time a thought enters into your mind about how ugly your past is and/or if anyone knew what you did and how they would ostracize you, stop and pick up the word of God. Quote scripture back to your thoughts. The Bible says in *2 Corinthians 10:5, "We are destroying speculations and every lofty thing that raises up against the knowledge of God and we are taking every thought captive to the obedience of Christ."*

Embarrassment

Guilt leads us to the third emotion that we feel due to our past and that is embarrassment. Embarrassment is defined as feeling self conscious, confused and having a loss of self confidence. Satan wants your past to make you feel embarrassed because he knows that you do not want anyone to know what you did. Many are scared that if their family or friends found out what they did, they would be cast into a negative light. You say to yourself, "I was a different person back then. I am not the same person now." You feel ashamed. The deceiver loves to use this emotion because this emotion causes you to feel poorly about yourself so that you separate yourself from others and become distant. Your family and friends are not sure if they have offended you, if you are ill or what the problem is. They just know that you are different. The bad thing is you would like to explain to them what is bothering you, but you can't; so you hold your past inside, safe, where no one can see it. What you fail to understand is that holding on to your past is toxic. Pretty soon, everything you do is contaminated because your past builds up a stench in you and no one wants to be around you because your negativity is so draining. Is that how you want to live your life? How can you expect to get pregnant with the negativity that is running through your veins?

God's Truth # 2
Romans 8:1 states, "Therefore there is now no condemnation for those who are in Christ Jesus. For the law of the Spirit of life in Christ Jesus has set you free from the law of sin and of death. For what the Law could not do, weak as it was through the flesh, God did: sending His own Son in the likeness of sinful flesh and as an offering for sin, He condemned sin in the flesh." If Satan is trying to destroy you by using your past, you need to start fighting back by using weapons that God has given us. Don't allow Satan to trick you into thinking that you are not getting pregnant because of your past. Start speaking this scripture back to him and follow it up with a little praise and worship, Satan cannot handle the Word or praise and worship.

Satan's Lie #3:
"Maybe you are not meant to be a mother, focus on your career. Climb the corporate ladder to success, forget about a family."

Analysis #3

Today, women have more educational opportunities and career options than ever before. As a result of this, society has planted the "career focused mindset" into their minds. This mindset is detrimental because it causes women to focus only on their career and nothing else. God's priority list places God first, family second and career third. However the "career focused mindset" distorts God's list and insists that our careers be placed above the family. Lie #3 is such a dangerous lie to fall prey to because the media perpetuates this stereotype of women doing everything men can do. Unfortunately, many women believe this myth. Don't be fooled, you can do most things that a man can do, but you can't do all of them. Why? Because God made man and woman differently, He did not make us the same. He gave men certain strengths and abilities that He did not give woman and vice versa. So before we compare ourselves to the creation that God made called man, we should make sure we are comparing apples to apples. Comparing and contrasting men and women is not apples to apples.

We teach our daughters to go to school and get an education, so they can go out and support themselves. We teach them everything about becoming independent and self-sufficient, but we don't teach them anything about becoming a joyful wife and mother. I believe teaching independence is a valuable lesson. After all, until God blesses them with a family, they will need to learn how to function dependently on God and independent of others. However, here's the crux of the argument. Many have been trying to conceive, only to later believe that they have failed. Thus, they decide to focus on their career. One might say "I know I perform well in my career. I receive bonuses and accolades from my superiors, so maybe I should just focus all of my energy on my career." Being successful in a career is fine, as long as it doesn't come before or interfere with family. Would God have you place your career ahead of your role as helpmate and caregiver to your family?

> Think about these questions and answer them truthfully to yourself:
> Do you think Satan is concerned about how well you progress in your career?
> Do you think he really wants you to succeed or be at the top of your field?"

If your answer is yes, then you need to analyze "Why?" Why does Satan want you to believe in your career so much? What does he gain by convincing you to forget about having a family?

I'm very glad you asked. I believe Satan has two reasons he wants you so focused on your career and not on your family: 1) He wants to prevent *Genesis 1:28, which says, "And God blessed them; and God said to them, Be fruitful and multiply and fill the earth."* God wants us to multiply His earth with children. You might say why is this so important? In God's Word, it says in *Psalms 78:5-7, "For He established testimony in Jacob and appointed a law in Israel, which He commanded our fathers that they should teach them to their children that the generation to come might know, even the children yet to be born, that they may arise and tell them to their children they should put their confidence in God and not forget the works of God, but keep His commandments."* God wants the knowledge of Him passed down to all generations, to all people and even to the ends of the earth. With more generations praising and glorifying God, He has more soldiers in His army. Now, don't get God wrong, He doesn't *need* you in His army. He can fight all battles by Himself, but He *wants* you in His army. I know what you are thinking, "But I've pursued getting pregnant and it's just not happening. That brings me to the conclusion that maybe I'm better at having a career than being a mother." Still, you must pursue conception. If Satan can convince you to focus on your career, instead of birthing more soldiers for Christ, then he accomplishes his goal of making sure no more Christian soldiers are born to fight against him and his army.

The second reason Satan wants you focused on your career is so he can destroy the harmony in a marriage between a husband and wife. If women are more focused on their careers than their home, then the Christian marriage suffers. You see, if the wife gets home later due to her workload or meetings, then dinner is late, the house is not clean, and pretty soon, chaos erupts in the home. Sure, the husband can pitch in and help, but the woman's focus is not on her family or her home, her mind is occupied with work-related items. Soon, the family is off of her list of important items. Daily, she picks up take-out for dinner and she fails to pay the bills on time. Eventually, her husband has noticed her absence physically and emotionally. As a result of this, he begins seeking advice from a co-worker about problems that he's having at work or at home, simply because his wife is unavailable to talk with him. She is too busy and to exhausted with her job. After time elapses, the communication between husband and wife is strained. Their discussions involve bills and other meaningless tasks that help the household run. Sooner than later, the husband is seeking his needs elsewhere while the wife is still performing her duties faithfully at work and constantly pleasing her boss. Next, the marriage is over, no children are produced and neither of them understands what happened. The deceiver wins again.

God never states in the Bible that a woman cannot have a career. In fact, *Proverbs 31* explains how to have a career and a balanced family life. The Bible says, "*So that her children and her husband rise up and call her blessed.*" Somehow, we have decided to climb the corporate ladder and make that our primary responsibility. We've become selfish by focusing on how we could progress to manager, director, then to vice president and so on. But we forget about the effect this has on our family. *Philippians 2:3-4 says, "Do nothing from selfishness or empty conceit, but with humility of mind let each of you regard one another as more important than himself; do not merely look out for your own personal interests, but also for the interests of others.*" If you are only focused on your career, then you are mainly looking out for yourself and not others. Have you thought about if you had a child, how that child would affect your career goals? Or would you continue your focus on career as you attempt to move up the corporate ladder—letting your child play by himself while you work a little late on that "important" project?

Have you replaced your husband with your boss? Do you spend more time looking good for your boss than you do for your husband? Could it be that you're not honoring your husband or his position over your life? Could this be the reason you don't have any children? If you've been placing your job above your husband, thus above your family, then maybe God hasn't blessed your womb because your priorities are out of order. I can't tell you that this is why you're having problems conceiving. But it's worth analyzing, especially if you spend more time at work than you do at home. I don't have a problem with women having careers; my problem is when women forget their role as a wife. When your career becomes the predominate factor in your life, then you have become engrossed and your priorities have become skewed. We have a God-given role in our marriages and it is not to wear the pants. In *1 Corinthians*

11:3, God established an order for us to follow, He says, *"But I want you to understand that Christ is the head of every man and the man is the head of a woman and God is the head of Christ."* God is first, then His Son, Jesus Christ, then man and then woman.

I hope this discussion has helped you to analyze your career and your home. I made the decision to place my career ahead of having a family after I could not conceive. Sure, I was successful, but after awhile, I became bored. God got my attention before my life, my happiness and my marriage were all in shambles.

God's Truth #3—*Psalms 119:133-134 states, "Order my footsteps in your word and do not let iniquity have dominion over me. Redeem me from the oppression of man, that I may keep your precepts."* **God wants you to allow Him to order your steps so that He can guide you in the direction He wants you to go. He says to keep His precepts, don't stray from what His Word says about you or to you. He wants us to realize that He has a plan for us and it's His plan not ours. Be patient and know that God will never leave us or forsake us, but that He will be with us always.**

Satan's Lie #4:
"If by chance I get pregnant, I probably won't be able to bring the baby to term. I will probably miscarry again."

Analysis #4:

Chance? Nothing happens in this world by chance. God is not a God of chance. Everything is designed and is purposed to happen because that's the way the Creator designed the world. God created everything and knows everything; so, nothing surprises Him. If God intends for you to get pregnant, you will get pregnant, and it will not be by chance. If you have had a miscarriage before, have you dealt with that loss and the pain it generated in your body and mind? Your past miscarriage or miscarriages does not necessary mean you are doomed to repeat the same fate once again. Miscarriages happen for a number of reasons, but it does not mean that you will always miscarry. Sometimes, God cleanses your body in order to prepare it for the new life He wants to bring forth. And you say, "If that's true, why does He have to clean it out that way?" I can't tell you that, but I do know it was not because of chance. *"His thoughts are not our thoughts and His ways are not our ways" (Isaiah 55:8).*

But you can believe He has His reasons and that's where faith comes into play. Job said, *"Though he slays me, yet shall I trust him". (Job 13:15)*

Miscarriages are hard on mothers because we get our hopes up and say, "This is it." We say to ourselves, "I am finally going to be a mommy." At two months pregnant, we buy little items for the baby—long before we even know the sex of the child. We memorize the due date and mark it on our calendars as a constant reminder. We are so excited and we want to tell everyone. Then something goes wrong and we blame God. We say, "Okay, I had a physical issue." A tumor was hindering the growth of the fetus. "Why didn't God shrink or remove the tumor, if He's all powerful?" Again, I can't answer that for you, but I can answer that for me.

I had a miscarriage in 2000 where a tumor was hindering the growth of the fetus. I believe that God allowed me to experience this pain so that I could minister to other women who have experienced or will experience that same pain. You see, God always has a reason for what He is doing in your life. He looks at our life as a complete picture. We only see pieces of our life day by day, but God sees the entire picture. He knows that everything we experience is for our good. He is sometimes developing our character, developing our faith, or sometimes teaching us patience. But whatever He is doing in our life is always for our good.

He never said this life would be a bed of roses. He said *there would be trials and tribulations throughout our days on this earth, (James 1:2).* For some of us, miscarriages are a part of our trials and tribulations. I have had two miscarriages and neither one was a pleasant experience. I ached in my body and in my heart because my womb that was once filled was now empty. I cried out to God, "Why?" I didn't find the answer to that question, until now. It was never just about me. Sure, God was and is concerned about me, but the miscarriages were never just about me. God is such an awesome God. In the midst of teaching me Godly principles for my life through the trial of infertility, He was also preparing a book about my struggle for women to read that would encourage, elevate and empower them in the Word of God during their season of infertility. *Revelations 19:6, states, "God is a voice of many waters."* This means He can use one word to bless many people. You hear one thing to bless your soul and another person hears something else that blesses theirs.

God's Truth #4: *Genesis 50:20 "As for you, you meant evil against me, but God meant it for good in order to bring about this present result, to preserve many people alive"* Remember that God always has a reason for what He does. Don't allow Satan to circumvent God's real intent for your miscarriage or burden. God loves us and wants to give us the desires of our hearts, but He has a plan and a time in which He wishes to reveal that plan. So trust, have faith and wait on Him for His answer. His word says in *Psalms 37:4 "Trust in the Lord and do good; dwell in the land and cultivate faithfulness. Delight yourself in the Lord; And He will give you the desires of your heart."*

I have shared with you some of the lies Satan told me as I walked on the journey of infertility. One way we can benefit God's kingdom is by multiplying the earth with offspring that are raised in the fear and admonition of Jesus Christ. We also benefit the kingdom by receiving the forgiveness of God for our past sins and maintaining a God-focused mentality instead of career-focused mentality. And finally, we stop believing in chance and start believing in God. *Proverbs 23:7 says, "For as a man thinks within, so is he"*. Develop a perspective of how God views who we are and what we do with our lives.

So the next time negative thoughts come in your mind, analyze where they are originating. Tell yourself, God loves me and I love me; and then ask, "Why am I feeling this way about myself and my circumstances?" God is a promoter of circumstances; therefore, let Him speak to your circumstances and begin to walk in what He says about you.

II

The Daddy and Daughter Relationship

7

God Loves His Daughters

1 John 5:18—We have come to know and have believed the love which God has for us. God is love, and the one who abides in love abides in God, and God abides in him.

It's no secret that most little girls, we all dream of being a mother someday. While we are young, we give special care and attention to our baby dolls in preparation for future motherhood. We demonstrate this care and concern by feeding our dolls, rocking them to sleep, dressing them and bathing them. We learn the art of nurturing from our own mothers, striving to duplicate this endearment with our dolls until that day when the role of nurturer can be fulfilled in our homes with our own children. Sure, playing with dolls seems like harmless play for a young girl, but it has lasting significance as we grow into adult women and begin to assume our roles as wife and mother. For some of us, giving birth to a baby has been a slow process, full of disappointment, anger and frustration. This slow process has caused all of our motherhood hopes and dreams to be dashed.

We all have seen the special bond between parents and children and we want to experience that bond as well. But as of yet, God has not blessed us with a baby and we are saddened because we believe that we may never be blessed with a child. For some of us, the special bond between a daddy and a daughter has never been experienced, but we have always longed for it. We know for a fact that a special bond does exist between a father and his daughter because even as adults we still yearn for it.

Perhaps, you are reading the title of this chapter and saying to yourself, "If only this were true in my life. What a joy it would be to conceive a child and present him/her as a gift to my husband. A child would make everything in our lives perfect. We would finally be considered a family after all this time. We could enjoy the sounds of laughter radiating throughout our home, while we continuously gather little toys left behind by our adventurous little one. Our family and our friends would be thrilled for us and all eyes would be fixated upon our new bundle of joy." You are probably thinking, "What I wouldn't give to be a mother? Oh, how I wish I could have a baby. I would love and cherish him/her like no other mother ever has. We would all be so happy."

Since you are thinking about motherhood, let's imagine that God has finally answered your prayers. You have a baby, a darling son who is so sweet and cuddly. He is healthy and happy and he has the perfect likeness of you and your husband. You love him so much and there is nothing that you would not do for him. He is priceless. This baby is all you ever wanted and he is in your arms right now. You are wondering about what he will grow up and become. You look at him and you want him to have everything, more than what you had as a child. You want him to have whatever his little heart desires. As you look at him, you know that you have to protect him from the evil of this world. You know he will endure disappointments and hurts, but you have decided that you will always be there for him because you are his mother and he needs you. Looking at him, you are amazed and overjoyed because he is finally here. You think about the good days ahead: his first cookie, trips to the park, his first little league game, and of course, his first girlfriend. You don't want to miss any major milestones.

But you are told that your son is special and that he has the power to save the world. But in order for the world to be saved, your son must die. Without his sacrificial offering, the world will perish and go to hell. The death of your son is the only way to save the world. Could you give up your <u>only child,</u> the one that has taken you so long to receive, knowing that He would be beaten, tortured and eventually killed?

Most people would say, "No, I can't do that." You might say, "This world is in trouble if they are waiting on me to give up my child." But the Bible states that "*God so loved the world that He gave His <u>only</u> begotten son, Jesus Christ" (John 3:16).* This illustration is to help you understand the love that God has for us and how He must have felt giving up His Son.

Let's break down the above verse a little bit. He gave His <u>only son</u> for the world. Many of us reading this book do not have children, but have a strong desire for children. Can you imagine yourself as God? Can you imagine having to give up your <u>only child</u>? Think about how much you want a child right now. God gave His Son for the world knowing that He would suffer persecution, feel loneliness, hatred, be viciously beaten and spat upon. But God made a decision to allow His Son to die. It was the only way that we, His people could be saved from eternal damnation. With all of the love He has for His Son, He loves us that much more because He sacrificed Him for us.

What kind of love does this? I can't imagine the ability of God to come to this decision and then actually follow through with it. Surely, if it were me, I would have tried to find other options. I would have pursued them first, before I turned my son over to people that hated, despised and would eventually kill him. The hurt and anguish that God must have felt had to be excruciating, unexplainable and unbearable.

But as hard as it must have been, He gave up His Son for us. Look in the mirror and ask yourself, "Was I worth it? Am I worth the suffering, the abuse, the physical pain that Christ felt for my sin? Have I proven today that I am worth it?" That answer is "NO," and you will never be able to prove that you are worth it. But you can humbly submit your life to God, recognizing His Son and the power of the Holy Spirit. He loves us so much that He freely decided to give up His most prized possession, so that we might be free. In the Bible, Romans 8 describes the road to salvation; it starts by believing that Jesus Christ died on a cross for your sins. It further states if you believe with your heart and confess with your mouth, then God saves you and you will reign in heaven with Him forever. It's just that simple. If you have not confessed Jesus as Lord and Savior over your life, take some time and do that right now. God wants to make you a joyful mother.

Going even deeper, have you made it your business to love God more than your desire to have a baby? Have you told Him that you want a baby, but even if He doesn't answer the way you want Him to, then His Will be done anyway? Have you submitted yourself and your womb to God? "God, if you choose not to answer my prayer, I will still praise you. I will still love you!"

Many of you may be thinking, I know that God loves me, but I have been waiting for years for God to bless my womb. God is the father of time and from God's vantage point, a minute is as a thousand years and a thousand years is as one minute. God wants us to understand that our thoughts are not His thoughts and our ways are not His ways. As you have read earlier in this book, God has a reason for everything He does. You may not have a baby right now because God is trying to show you His love or deeper issues that reside in you or maybe complete dependence on Him. Whatever the reason, God wants you first and foremost to understand the measure of love that He has for you. Perhaps one way to get your attention focused on His love is to use the trial of infertility.

The qualities and characteristics that God exhibits towards us should be the same ones we exhibit toward our children. I know what you are thinking, "But I don't have any children." While that is true now, you must start thinking like a joyful mother in preparation for the child that God will give you.

God tells us He loves us, wants to spend time with us and shows us daily of His love for us. How are you demonstrating your love for a child? Do you have any relatives or friends with children? Have you communicated to them that you love them? Do you spend any time with them and do you show them that you love and care for them? When is the last time you offered to baby-sit someone's child or take the child for the afternoon to give another mom a break? How many moms, especially single moms, do you know that could use a couple of hours of alone time one evening or on the weekend? Or, if you don't know anyone with kids, when is the last time you visited an orphanage or volunteered at a women's shelter? Have you ever spent time with a child by reading a book and/or working on a puzzle with them?

There are children everywhere who need love and attention. Have you thought of becoming a foster parent to provide love to children who are scared and stuck in the system? The Bible also says when you do this to the least of them, you do it unto me *(Matthew 18:5)*. Or have you spent your time, day in and day out, crying and worrying about why you don't have a child?

There is a principle in the Bible called seed time and harvest time and it is mostly used to explain the concept of tithing. However, it can be used to understand other principles as well. Seed time and harvest time from a farming perspective means that farmers prepare the ground by tilling the soil and watering it. When the ground is ready, farmers take seed, maybe tomato, or onion or whatever seed they wanted to spring forth. They plant the seed in the ground and wait for the seed to blossom into plants with vegetation on them. Later, the farmers collect their harvest and sell or eat it. By giving the soil its' seed, the farmer is able to receive the harvest based on the type of seed he sowed. Thus, if a farmer wants corn, he wouldn't sow wheat.

Seed Time/Harvest Time Principle

Now, how does this concept help me while I am waiting for God to bless me with a child? Maybe you are waiting on a child, but you have not sown anything to receive a child. What have you planted or sown with regard to children? Make it a point to reread the above paragraph and start planting seeds so you can begin reaping the benefits of a being a joyful mother.

8

God Protects His Daughters

1 Peter 1:5—....who are protected by the power of God through faith.......

Since we know how much God loves us, it will stand to reason that He wants to protect us from negative environments, people and situations, including those situations we cause ourselves. This doesn't mean that God will not allow harm to come our way. But rather, He allows what seems to be harmful in order that we gain something greater. In this, He also protects us. He could allow all kinds of travesties to come our way, all at one time. Instead, He only allows some challenges to come our way and He gives us the strength to get through them.

Sometimes, He has to protect us from things that we want like new jobs, new relationships, finances, etc. Sometimes, we see these things as good, but God sees their true nature and knows that they will cause us more harm than good. What may be good for one person, may not be good for another because God has made each one of us differently. We are all unique in that your experiences, your desires, and your gifts are different than mine. I thank God that He does not treat us all the same because we are different and we have different needs that only He can fill. And as a result of our uniqueness, He protects us in different ways as well. There are some things that I need protection from that you may not and then there are situations that we all need protection from and God faithfully protects.

For example, in *Luke 11:11-13*, a little boy sees an egg and asks his father to give it to him. The father denies his request and the boy becomes upset. The boy saw the egg as something good for him to eat and he was confused as to why his father would deny him food. But what the little boy could not see was what he thought was an egg was not an egg at all. In reality, it was a white scorpion curled up in the shape of an egg. The father would not give his son something that would harm him, even though the boy desperately wanted it. Like the father of this story, our Heavenly Father promises to *protect you from dangers seen and unseen*". He never leaves us nor forsakes us and He is always there for us. Even when we do not deserve His mercy and grace, He continues to give chance after chance. We continue to fail, but He still never abandons us.

Sometimes, God needs to protect us from ourselves. You might ask yourself "Why would God need to protect me from myself?" After all, "I love myself and I would never intentionally do anything to hurt me." And for some of us, this statement is true. We would never do anything intentional to hurt ourselves, but what about the things we do that are unintentional. You say, "Kim, what do you mean?" I mean, our thoughts can hurt us and God protects us from our thoughts. Did you know that negative thoughts can sometimes harm you more than physical pain? Sometimes, we allow ourselves to see only the negative about ourselves and our situation.

Let me give you an example of what I am talking about. "I am so tired of trying to get pregnant; I'll never have a baby. I'm such a failure. Why did God put me on this earth if I can't even give birth? I can't even do what the Bible says I am supposed to do." Maybe you're never thought these thoughts, but I have. *The Bible says in Psalms 94:11, "The Lord knows the thoughts of man."*

Because God knows our thoughts, He takes steps to protect us from those thoughts. He does this by sending someone our way with an encouraging word, or He may speak to us while we are reading, driving or just sitting quietly. God doesn't want us to focus on our present condition. He wants us to admit our desires, but to control our negative thoughts. *The Bible says in Matthew 15:19, "For out of the heart come evil thoughts...and verse 20 says, "These are the things which defile man."* Defile means to make filthy or unclean. If you allow yourself to focus on negative thoughts, these thoughts will consume you as you speak them to others and give birth to a negative reality. *Proverbs 23:7 says "For as a man thinks within himself, so he is." The Bible goes on to say in Proverbs 18:21, "Death and life are in the power of the tongue, and those who live it will eat its fruit."* **Do you realize what you are doing? If you speak words of defeat over your body and its ability to reproduce, the power of your tongue produces death in your womb.** Think about that. You might not be pregnant right now because the thoughts from your heart have turned into words cast out from your mouth and caused a curse over your body. You have said, "I'll never get pregnant," and now your words have caused it to be so.

Did you ever think that your words could have so much power? Well, God says they do. Think back to your thoughts and how those thoughts have materialized into words. That's why you must read the Bible and pay attention to its instruction. *In 2 Corinthians 10:5, "We are taking every thought captive to the obedience of Christ."* This means every thought must be examined before it is conceived in your heart and cast out of your mouth. Have you been cursing yourself? Thank God, He stops us and reminds us of His goodness. He always wants to protect us from ourselves, our thoughts, our words.

That's why we must operate in faith. Faith is the key to living a fulfilled life. Without faith in God, we are lost and subject to the evil that invades our thoughts and fills this world. The next time a negative thought comes before you, see yourself as God sees you. He says in *Romans 8:37, "But in all these things, we overwhelmingly conquer through Him, who loved us."* So stand firm and know that God protects you from everything, even yourself.

Seed Time/Harvest Time Principle

You may not be able to protect all children, but you should pray for their protection. If you are asking which children should you pray for, pray for children that you know as well as those you don't know. But be specific in your prayer; pray for the protection of all the children that have been abducted, all children in schools, all children in abusive family situations, homeless children and those in foster care.

9

God Provides For His Daughters

In Philippians, 4:19, it says that God will supply all your needs according to His riches in glory in Christ Jesus".

What a wonderful feeling it is to know that God provides for our every need whether we ask Him to or not. For most of us, the most pressing need that we have right now is the need to have a baby. We should examine...is that a need or a desire? A need is the something that you are unable to do without. Whereas, a desire is a longing, a wanting or a strong wish. Material needs are things in your life that you are desperate to have (i.e. food, shelter, clothing, reliable transportation, etc.) Material desires are those things that you would like to have, but can do without (i.e. designer clothes, jewelry, spa packages, BMW, etc.) God provides for both our needs and desires based upon His sovereign will. But what about those nonmaterial things like physical wellness and emotional completeness? These can be construed as needs or desires as well. Material/nonmaterial needs and desires are received through Jesus Christ's nurturing power. You might classify having a baby as a need for you in your life. That's fine because only you know what is a need or a desire for you. Just so you know, a baby was a need for me, too. If we believe in God's word, then we must believe that He and only He can supply all of our needs and desires and more.

How does He meet these needs? God provides for us by nurturing us. There are many ways that God nurtures us, but let's focus on three. They are: through prayer, reading God's word and meditation on His word. Through these, God nurtures us just like you would nurture a baby. Sure, a baby has physical needs: feeding, changing their diaper and bathing, but a baby also has emotional needs that also must be nurtured.

Babies love to be cuddled close to their mother because mothers provide that soothing sense of calm and peace. Oftentimes, when babies are crying and there is nothing wrong with them, they are comforted just by their mother picking them up. They know she is there to provide for all of their needs, even in times of fussiness and anxiety. Think about a mother putting her baby to sleep, she calms the baby by stroking the baby's arm or hair. That baby receives that touch of love and is changed forever because he knows that touch is born from genuine love and concern for his well-being. Oftentimes, the mother places the baby's head on her heart because it is familiar and is the first sound they hear. Instantly, the bond is formed, the baby looks to the mother and wants the mother for everything. There is something so special about the love between a mother and child. Why do you think most children call for their mommies when they are hurt and/or when they have accomplished an important task? They know that mommy can make it all better and in turn they feel her love in the process. That bond between mother and child is so strong, that no matter what, a child always loves his/her mother and vice versa. I am not saying that fathers cannot love and make a baby feel safe and secure. They can, but usually the baby prefers the mother to accomplish this goal. Dad's role becomes stronger later especially in the pre-teen and teen years and beyond. As an adult, this makes me think, "What does it feel like for a baby to be cuddled close to his mother and feel like this is the best place in the world to be?" Imagine the calm, quiet and content feeling that must be for a child. Wouldn't it be nice to have that feeling again? Well, that feeling can be relived over and over, if we allow God to nurture us.

One way we can allow God to nurture us is through prayer. *Hebrews 4:16 states, "To come boldly to the throne of grace, so that you may receive mercy and find grace to help in time of need."* Prayer is direct communication with the Father and as the scripture states, we should not be shy to approach God, but we are to approach Him boldly. Prayer allows us to explain our thoughts, worries and fears to God, just as a child would to his father or the way you would to a close friend. Talking to God through prayer is healing within itself because it allows us to get concerns and problems out into the open with God. Not that He does not already know them, but this gateway of prayer allows us to clear our conscience and "be real" with God, truly discussing our hurts, disappointments and fears about trying to conceive. Prayer also allows the burden of our problems to shift from us carrying them to God carrying them.

The Bible says in Matthew 11:28-29, "Come to Me, all who are weary and heavy-laden and I will give you rest. Take my yoke upon you and learn from Me, for I am gentle and humble in heart and you will find rest for your souls. For My yoke is easy and My burden is light." This is a comforting scripture for many of you right now because you are experiencing emptiness, confusion and depression. Many of you are so weary from the long struggle of trying to conceive that all you know is a life of ups and downs, highs and lows filled with constant disappointment. That means you are weary. Weariness makes you tired and causes you to lack hope and eventually stop believing that God can really bless you with a baby. With weariness comes feelings of heavy-ladeness. You've carried this burden so long that it is now a part of you and it seems as though it is never going to end. As a result, your heart is heavy and the burden is heavy and sometimes it feels as though you can't place one foot in front of the other.

Stop carrying this burden by yourself. Instead, pick it up and unload it on the Father. We have a God who is more than capable and able to carry every burden. Let Him carry it! Thank God, this verse tells us, it's OK to be disappointed and disgusted with your circumstance. In fact, it's normal, but instead of trying to handle the problems yourself, take them to God and let Him handle them. All He wants you to do is come to Him. He tells us that His yoke is easy and His burden is light. What better advice could we receive and what better comfort could God provide for us? God listens to our prayers and looks at our hearts. Prayer is seen by God as an act of dependence on Him and is a powerful tool because it activates His power within us. When we pray to God, we are acknowledging that we need Him, trust Him and depend on Him to help us, advise us and guide us. It demonstrates to God that we are not actively pursuing our lives independent of Him. God sees that we value Him and what He thinks about us. And we know that whatever our prayers entail, He has the power to answer them.

Did you know that a lack of emotional completeness can affect your physical well-being which can cause you to _not_ conceive? Is your emotional incompleteness preventing your womb from being filled? If this is the case, talk to God. He so desires for us to talk to Him, trust Him and love Him. We need prayer in our lives on a daily basis. We are told throughout the Bible that Jesus prayed to God constantly. We need to follow Jesus' example of praying without ceasing. Our day should not start until we talk to our Heavenly Father. After all, He has given us *"each day our daily bread"*. If you want a baby, talk to God. Tell Him if you think it's unfair for everyone else to have a baby and not you. He is your Father; so you must honor Him, but explain to Him how you feel.

He wants to hear it from you. Tell Him that you're ready to have children. I can't promise you that He'll answer the way you want Him to or even when you want Him to, but He will answer. God always answers prayers with Yes, No or Wait. Begin building your relationship with God and let God nurture you through prayer. *The Bible in 2 Chronicles 7:14 says, "If my people who are called by my name will humble themselves and pray and seek my face and turn from their wicked ways, then I will hear from heaven, and I will forgive their sin and I will heal their land".* God is waiting on you to humble yourself, pray and seek Him. Allow Him to heal you. If you have miscarried or had an ectopical pregnancy, pray for Him to heal your body and your heart from your loss. If there is sin in your life, which we all have sinned, confess that sin and ask for the strength not to sin and grieve Him anymore. Tell Him you believe in His sacrificial offering and thank Him for it. Just talk to Him and let your heart lead you. *The Bible says, "If you draw close to Him, He will draw closer to you." Philippians 4:6 says, "Be anxious for nothing, but in everything through prayer and supplication let your requests be known to God".* It's really up to you. But, if you want to feel the safe and secure feeling that a baby feels when it is nestled up against it's mother, you must humble yourself and pray with the confidence that God will provide that same comfort for you.

Another way that God nurtures us is by the reading of His Word. This type of spiritual nurturing is a vital component in developing and maintaining a relationship with God. How can you grow and cultivate your spirit without the Word of God? Throughout this book, you have seen the Bible quoted and referenced. However, I could not quote it or reference it if I had never read it. You need to read the Bible and follow its illustrations and instructions realizing that every situational question in life is answered in this one book. *In John 1:1, the Bible says, "In the beginning was the Word and the Word was with God and the Word was God."* How many of us have taken the time to read what God's Word says about children or barrenness? How can we say we know God if we have not taken time to read His Word? It's the instruction manual for our lives. If all our questions are answered in this book, why aren't we reading it?

We don't read the Bible or pay enough attention to it because we don't truly believe that all of life's questions are answered in it. Sure we believe it is important, but we don't really think it can help us with this problem. Some of us believe the Word is a group of great stories about Christ and many are comforting, but they don't really relate to the issues here today. Some believe that the Bible deals with ancient issues and was perfect for that time, but is irrelevant for modern day issues. After all, we have new technology, environmental issues and other social issues that are entirely different from those dealt with in biblical times. And as a result of this attitude, the Bible couldn't possibly help me with the problems that I am facing right now. Wrong! The Bible addresses all problems, even modern day ones, because the Word is God. The Bible says the word is sharper than any two-edged sword. This "ancient" book can help you get through this "modern" trial by providing encouragement and knowledge. It demonstrates how God feels and relates to His children. If some of us were really truthful about our thoughts concerning the Bible, we may even question God's true existence. We see tragedies such as 911 and the tsunami in Asia and we don't really see how a living God could allow these travesties to ever happen. Now, we wouldn't admit it and we sure wouldn't say it publicly, but the thought is there.

Don't you know God knows your true thoughts about His Word and about Him? What you're trying to hide is made completely visible to the Father. (Remember the "all knowing" omniscient person when you maintain this negative attitude and allow it to fester, denying the power of God, Jesus Christ, and the Holy Spirit.) Now, don't get me wrong, just because you are thinking in this manner does not hinder or negate God's power over His creation. You are just negating His power within your life. If you actually read the Bible, you will find that the same issues we face today were faced in biblical times and God provided an answer through His Word. Just pick up the Bible and research any issue and you will find it covered in the Holy Word. Infertility has been an issue since the beginning of time. There are many stories and references in the Bible to barrenness and how God answers and we'll cover those stories throughout this book.

We have seen that God nurtures through prayer and the reading of His Word. Now, let's look at meditation. Meditation is another way God spiritually nurtures us. This form of spiritual nurturing is key because it involves hearing from God. Life has so many twists and turns. There is always something attempting to distract us from our goal. That's why it's important to sit down quietly with God's Word and listen to how it applies to your situation. For example, let's look at some typical distractions at work, we have promotion concerns, a need for more money, a decision to change careers, corporate restructuring of the company, layoffs, personality conflicts with co-workers, bosses, vendors, clients, etc.,—and that's just work.

As you can see, life is so noisy and filled with distractions that meditation is something that you will have to exert extra energy to accomplish it. That's only if your heart truly wants to hear from God. Combine the work distractions with life's other distractions and you will find there seems to be very little time to meditate. Why do we let all of these distractions take priority in our lives? One reason is because God is not truly first in our lives. We don't deny Christ as Lord and we don't deny the power of His Word. It's just not the first thing on our list. Unfortunately for us, it is at the bottom. If we are honest with ourselves, the truth is, we seek the other agenda first and if that doesn't go according to our plans then we seek God. *The Bible says in Matthew 6:33, "Seek ye first the kingdom of God and His righteousness and all these things will be added to you."*

Just like having a baby, most of us have tried everything else: ovulation testing, counting the days, fertility drugs and now we are trying God. Why didn't we start with God first? As I'm speaking to you, I speak to myself. How many times have we looked to the advice of others on how to get pregnant, not thinking to ask God first? Please tell me what's wrong with us? Some of us have been in church all of our lives and know to seek God first, but we routinely seek Him last. What's our problem? As *Isaiah 40 says "Do you not know or have you not heard? The Everlasting God, the Lord, the Creator of the ends of the earth does not become weary or tired. His understanding is inscrutable."* When we begin to meditate on God's Word, to ask His advice and to trust Him to work our situation out for us, He hears us and answers.

While I was trying to get pregnant, I asked everyone for advice. I received information from friends about how to make love in order for the sperm to have an easier passageway to the egg. I read books on how to get pregnant fast. I prayed to God to let me conceive, but I never asked God for His advice. Instead of talking to God constantly about why you are not pregnant, find verses in the Bible that relate to barrenness and study what God was trying to teach that individual. In addition to this, read the verses, meditate on the verses and listen to what He has to say about them for you. The definition of barrenness is to be without child, sterile, that which cannot produce offspring.

Think about the concept of barrenness and meditate on this. Are there areas in your life that are barren? Examine yourself and listen to what the Lord says about those areas in your life. He likes to utilize our experiences and challenges in order to teach us something about ourselves. Maybe, you won't receive a blessing of a baby until you have fully examined yourself and made some changes.

In your examination of barrenness, focus on two factors: 1) What am I without? Is the answer to this question faith in God, love for my fellow man, true contentment or etc.? You have to determine for yourself what you are lacking? Or 2) What is it I need to be without? Is your answer to this question, hatred toward a co-worker or family member, jealously of a friend getting a new house or good husband? Meditate on this concept and really search your soul for the answers to the above questions. Most importantly, pray that God will guide you to the correct answers for your life. You might say, "Well I have done this, so what's my next step?" Your next step is to flourish in the Lord while you wait on His answer. If there are areas in your life that do not represent Christ-like qualities or the true fruit of the Spirit, then remove them and replace them with *love, joy, peace, patience, kindness, goodness, faithfulness, gentleness, and self control" (Galatians 5:22-23).* Again, God will often keep blessings from us until we make necessary changes. A lot of us have created some messed up lives by poorly handling a situation or various situations that have come up. (A very wise person once said, "God won't bless a mess." In other words, we need to correct some of our deficiencies, so we're free to receive all the blessing God has in store for us.)

Seed Time/Harvest Time Principle

What can you do in your current position to bless children? We all have friends and family with children. Spend some time and encourage them to pray, read their Bibles and meditate on God's Word. In addition to this, there are many children in poverty stricken areas of the community that are in need of toys and clothing at Christmas, as well as extra money for school field trips and activities. You could even sow seeds into the lives of children that are overseas by providing a small monthly amount of money to sponsor a child who needs food, water and clothing.

10

God Speaks to His Daughters

Deuteronomy 5:24—…we have heard His voice from the midst of the fire; we have seen today that God speaks with man…

The Word says in *Matthew 7:7, "Ask and it will be given to you; seek, and you will find; knock, and it will be opened to you".* How many times have we approached a problem without God? How many times can we say we prayed to God and listened to hear His response? Or have you decided ahead of time, I'll handle this problem myself or maybe it will just work itself out? God hears our audible and inaudible explanations about how we're going to handle our problems with or without Him. God wants us to verbally request our needs and desires to Him. He enjoys the interaction that we have with Him and when we submit ourselves to Him, we illustrate our dependence on Him. He wants to be our Father and our Friend, God wants to talk with us, but that cannot happen unless we talk and listen to Him daily.

Imagine that you have a teenage daughter and she is experiencing so many new thoughts and feelings in this new time in her life called adolescence. As her mother, you want to talk to her about everything she is feeling and thinking, but she will not talk to you. She is encountering girls who talk about sex, concerns about their appearance and certain types of clothing. She even has an interest in a young man, about which you know nothing. Your daughter has questions about sex, but prefers to receive answers from her girlfriends who have already experimented with sex, instead of talking to you. As her mother, you want to talk and listen to her concerns so that you can help guide her into making the right decisions, but she refuses to come to you for advice. As a matter of fact, she doesn't think you know very much about her issues or what she may be feeling or going through. She has become secretive and she completely shuts you out.

Do you think God feels this way? Each day is a new day for every one of us. It's full of experiences and challenges that we have not faced before. God is waiting for us to talk to Him, so He can guide us in making the right decisions and direct us on the right life path; but, we have shut Him out just like the teenager in the example above.

The Bible says in 1 Peter 5:7, "Cast all your cares upon Him for He cares for you."

So we know He cares for us, He tells us so; but, we don't feel the need to listen to God because we think, "God, I know how you would tell me to handle this problem, but I have to take care of this myself."

The skill of listening involves hearing what someone else is saying to you. In order to listen to God, you must be open to hear what is being said to you and that can only happen if you have a relationship with Him. God does not communicate with everyone the same way. When you call yourself a daughter of Christ, there should be a relationship with Him and you hear from God. For example, your mother may tell you certain things to help you, her daughter that she might not tell a stranger. Why? Your mother has your best interest at heart because she loves you. Your mother may not feel obligated to give another young lady that same advice, even though it will help her, because that young lady doesn't have the same relationship.

Matthew 11:25, says, "I praise you, Father Lord of heaven and earth that You have hidden these things from the wise and intelligent and have revealed them to infants." If you have a relationship with Him, He will reveal things to you that He may not reveal to your neighbor. Perhaps, this is not your issue; maybe you have talked to God and are waiting for His answers. You have decided to quiet yourself and listen to God's plan and purpose for your life and the life of your family. If so, congratulations. You are now developing a relationship with the Father. The more conversations you have with Him and the more you listen to Him speak, the better off your life will be.

Let's discuss the ways God has spoken to me in my life, but realize, you can't limit God. He has His own way of speaking to each one of us. God speaks to me in many different ways, but there are four main ways He speaks: 1) white doves; 2) people; 3) through His Word, prayer and mediation; and 4) physical objects—books.

One way He speaks to me is through His creation, God uses doves to speak to me by comforting me and confirming decisions that I believe God has led me to make. God started using this method in 1998 around the same time I got married.

In 1998, exactly seven days after I was married, my new husband and I were involved in a bad car accident that took me off of work for six weeks. I had a borderline fracture to my right arm, cuts on my legs and a concussion. At that time, I worked for a company where I was quite unhappy with my position; but, I did have a job and I was thankful. I saw limited upward movement in the company for myself and the position required some travel. The travel was a problem because I was newly married and my spouse's position also required him to travel. After I returned to work from my injury, I was issued a new laptop. The laptop worked fine until one day I had a problem with my laptop. I could not get it to work.

Let me explain what was happening. I would open the laptop and a white bird would fly across the screen continuously. I called my husband and told him what was going on. He told me to bring the computer home and he would look at it and try to fix it. I got home later that night and my husband examined the computer, but he could not figure out what was wrong. The computer would not start up and we could not turn it off. All we did was open up the laptop and there was the white bird flying across the screen. So, I contacted the Information technology department about this problem and they stated that they had never seen or heard of anything like this before. Because the occurrence was so confusing, the company went as far as to accuse me of sabotaging and/or tampering with the laptop. I remained calm, but explained that all I did was open the laptop in order to complete my work; I had not tampered with it at all. As a matter of fact, I know very little about computers and would not know how to sabotage one.

I continued trying to figure out why this white bird was flying on my screen. They told me to hold on to it and they would try to ship me another one.

I continued to try to stop the bird, but to no avail. While I had the computer, I prayed my normal prayers and God made it abundantly clear that the dove was a sign. He was speaking to me through these white doves. Because of my travel and unhappiness with the job, this attitude of discontent spilled into my marriage. The friction had become so bad that my husband told me that I could either submit my resignation or he would do it for me. He could not stand the discontent that was in our home. So I quit.

My resignation was submitted with reluctance. You see, I had just gotten married a couple of months earlier and I was not ready to trust and rely solely on my husband to be the provider, but I had no choice; I had to surrender my will for God's will.

Don't get me wrong, I had other signs that showed me that I needed to quit, but I ignored them. However, this one I could not ignore. My job caused me great stress which in turn, caused me to neglect my marriage. Till this day, God shows me Himself through white doves. Sometimes they fly over me while I'm driving or when I look out of the window, they're sitting in the yard. White doves are God's way of reminding me that He is always with me. When I see them, I smile. I feel Him near me. Right now, November 15, 2004, I am at the library writing this book and looking out a window. There are 14 white doves sitting on top of the pier by the water. That tells me, I'm doing exactly what God wants me to do which is to write this book. Thank You Lord and I Love You, too!

The goal of speaking and listening to God is to do what He tells us to do. For many of us, we speak to God and even hear from God, but, we fail to do what He's asked us to do.

What happens when you have heard from God, but you choose not to follow his instructions? For example, let's say God has told you that you will conceive and have a baby from your womb; however, you have not experienced it yet, so you're getting a little anxious. In order to help God out with His promise, you decide to start on fertility drugs or invitro fertilization. My question to you is, "Are you listening and following what God has spoken for your life or are you doing it yourself?"

I'm not against fertility drugs or invitro fertilization. In fact, I too have used fertility drugs, but God did not tell me to do so. I did it on my own. And as a result of me handling this problem myself, God refused to bless my womb. Now, if God is instructing you to use fertility drugs or invitro fertilization, then by all means, you should comply with His wishes; but, I believe if God spoke heaven and earth into being, then I am sure He can speak to your womb and it be filled with your baby. God does not need our help. He is omnipotent, which means all powerful. The Bible says the power of heaven and earth are in His hands and it states in *Hebrews 1:3*, *".... He upholds all things by the word of His power."* The Bible further states in *Mark 4.41*, *"Who then is this, that even the wind and the sea obey Him."* So, all God has to do is speak and the winds and waters obey Him.

During this trial in your life, you have to become totally dependent on Him for your breakthrough. If you have taken matters into your own hands, God will let you handle it. If God says, you will give birth to a baby, then you must believe that you will give birth to a baby. You must be patient and have faith in what God has spoken to you, and most importantly, refrain from helping Him out. *James 1: 6-7 says, "If you cannot trust and believe in what God says then we should not expect anything from God."*

I realize this statement is a tough pill to swallow, but God does not play around with His trust and faith. He has given up everything for us, the very least we can do is trust Him and His Word. His word will do for us exactly what it says it will do. In our society with all of its new innovations and technology, sometimes modern science wants to play God. Sure, it's great to take advantage of the knowledge and expertise that God has given scientists. The problem occurs when scientists refuse to give God credit for the blessing of that knowledge and expertise. It's not science, <u>it is God </u>and God gave man science. You should not hear a mother say that invitro is the best thing that ever happened to her. I have heard women say that and it saddens my heart because they have confused science with giving life. Instead, she should say because of God and His infinite wisdom in placing this knowledge and ability into scientists, God is the best thing that happened to her. It is always God who gives life.

Let me give you an example. I know a lady who was diagnosed with ovarian cancer and the doctors had to take one of her ovaries, leaving her with just one. She endured painful treatment (radiation and/or chemo), but her husband is a strong man of faith and they desired to have children, however, with one ovary, the odds were stacked against them. Her husband said that he believed that God told him to marry his wife and they would have children together. Well, the doctors said the chances of her having a baby were slim to none with one ovary. Today, they have five beautiful children, all produced from that one ovary. Look at what God did! He took a barely functioning ovary and blessed it abundantly. The fruit of that blessing is not one, but five healthy children. Now, is God good or what!

You have to determine for yourself, "How does God speak to you?"

11

God Forgives His Daughters

1John 1:9—If we confess our sins, He is faithful and righteous to forgive us our sins and to cleanse us from all unrighteousness.

Psalms 79:9 states, "Help us, O God our salvation for the glory of Your name; And deliver us and forgive our sins for Your name's sake." Did you know that God forgives you even when you commit wrongs against Him? God is such a loving, patient and kind God that He forgives us of our sins. I know what you are thinking, "If God is so loving and powerful, then why won't He bless my womb. This would seem a little feat for an all-knowing ever-present and all powerful God. Why hasn't He done it?" Perhaps, you have been holding a grudge against God because He has not blessed you with a baby. You could be holding a grudge and not even know it. Ask yourself, "Am I mad at God because He has not answered my prayer?" Maybe you need to ask Him to forgive you for how you have treated Him? Have you given Him the honor that He deserves and so is worthy to receive? He forgives us even when we are mad and blame Him for our circumstances. If you are upset with or even mad at God, please confess that right now for He is faithful to forgive. Let Him pour His precious love on you and shower you with His grace. He is waiting for you to forgive Him. God loves you and has a perfect plan for your life. And, His plan is full of bountiful blessings, but He will not move forward to give it to you as long as you do not have forgiveness in your heart.

Sometimes, we need to get things right with God before He blesses us. Sometimes, our perspective is tainted because we look at our situation mainly by what we see and what we think, not by what God's Word says. Allow God to cleanse you of past thoughts and hurts for He is a loving and forgiving God who is open and willing to hear from you; however, you must take the first step by asking. Show Him that you are His daughter who loves Him and wants to return back to Him. Go to Him now.

When we choose not to forgive it, only hurts us. It does not hurt God. Sure, He has compassion for you, but He's not hurt. You know how we treat those with whom we disagree; we withdraw. We purposely hold back some of ourselves from that person.

Let me give you an example, your fifth grade little boy comes home with a note regarding his bad behavior at school. He's supposed to have you sign it and return it back to the school. Instead, he signs it himself and the teacher calls you because she is suspicious of the signature. You explain to her that you did not see the note, nor did you sign the note. Later on that evening, when your son gets home from soccer practice, you ask him about the note from the teacher. He confesses that he did not show you the note and that he forged your signature. As a result of his dishonesty, you ground him. Your son is deeply upset because his friend is having a really cool birthday party during the time he is grounded. In turn, he withdraws from you. For several days, he's upset and only gives you yes or no answers to your questions. When he comes home from school, he spends most of his time in his room because he does not want to be around you. In essence, he has a grudge against you and, therefore, wants to spend little or no time with you.

Is this your behavior toward God because He hasn't blessed you with a child? I hope not. Remember, we are the created and He is the creator. A lot of times, we want to make our relationship with God mimic our earthly relationships. Although, we can't do that, God is not like anyone else. We have to treat Him according to His sovereignty. He simply won't allow anything else. He is a Spiritual Being, majestic by nature and He deserves the highest honor and respect. Can you imagine what life would be like for us if God held a grudge against us? Just think, if the King of Kings decided to hold His grace and mercy from us because He was mad at us? You think your situation is bleak now; you have no idea what your life would be like if God turned His back and left you. That's what we do to people who anger or mistreat us. We act as if they do not exist, just like the fifth grader in the previous example. If God did this to us, we would have no direction, no guidance, no protection, no provision and most importantly—no love. Aren't you glad that God continues to love and forgive even when we have held a grudge against Him?

God not only forgives you for your sins, He forgives others for their sins. Before we go forward, I want you to know that sin is sin to God. There are not degrees of sin in God's sight; one sin is no greater than another. *Romans 3:23* clearly states, *".....for all have sinned and fall short of the glory of God."* We often want to judge sin on our own scale. We think if you commit murder that is a bigger sin than if you lie. It is not in God's sight, both are considered sin.

As I was asking for forgiveness for my own sins, it occurred to me, what about all the people who have sinned against God by harming children. *The Bible says, "whatever you do to the least of these my little children, you do unto to me."* I know that if they confess Jesus Christ as their Lord and Savior that He forgives their sins. *The Bible says in Acts 10:34, that "God is no respecter of persons,"* so what He does for me, He will do the same for you. As I was contemplating the many social wrongs, empty people and evil desires that seem to run rampant and harm many children, God reminded me of how He sees them. Look with me at our world today and the evil that is done toward children:

I see:

In parts of Africa, men with AIDS rape young girls and babies because a witch doctor told them that sleeping with a virgin would cleanse their bodies of the disease called AIDS.

Children in foster care where some foster care parents abuse, neglect and ridicule them because they are an extra responsibility.

In Washington, D.C., some mothers give birth to children and leave them in the hospital to be wards of the state. They are called border babies. Some are born addicted to drugs or diagnosed with HIV.

Many children have been physically abused and/or sexually abused. For example, children who have cigarette holes burned on their arms and legs, or a child who is starving to death and locked in a closet as a form of punishment; Mothers who choose to prostitute their bodies for drugs while their toddlers and babies are left at home alone fending for themselves and their siblings; Mothers who drown and mutilate their children, stating that God told them to do it.

These are just a few examples I've pulled from various headline stories. I could not possibly list them all. But amazingly God loves these mothers the same as He loves us. Yet there are mothers out there who just want the chance to be a mother while there are those that throw their children away or destroy them. *John 3:16-18, For God so loved the world that He gave His only begotten Son, that whoever believes in Him shall not perish, but have eternal life. For God did not send his son into the world to judge the world, but that the world might be saved through Him. He who believes in Him is not judged...."* God so loved the world means God loved everyone and everything in the world.

Seed Time/Harvest Time

Is there someone out there that you need to forgive? If so, take some time to go to that person and forgive them, as well as seek their forgiveness. Unforgiveness is like poison in your veins that affects every part of your life. Sow a seed of forgiveness and reap God's abundant forgiveness.

12

God Disciplines and Rewards His Daughters

Revelation 3:19 Those whom I love, I reprove and discipline...
Psalms 58:11—Surely there is a reward for the righteous.

God does not punish us; however, He will discipline us by allowing us to experience some of the consequences of our actions. But unlike us, God does not hold a grudge. Some of us have grudges against people that have been going on for years. God truly forgives and forgets. We're the ones that feel the need to remind Him of all of the evil things we've done in our past.

Children obey and listen to their parents. Children also learn from their parents. Could it be that God has not blessed you with a child because you have not acted as His child? Have you been respectful of what God is doing in your life or have you rebelled and decided that you're going to do your own thing? Thank God, He is patient and forgiving. He continues to give us chance after chance to change our behavior and conform to his image.

Remember when you were a child and your mother asked you not to do something, but you did it anyway? What happened? I'm sure she talked to you sternly, privileges were taken away from you or you were spanked. God's response is similar to our parents because He sets the model for parenting. If we truly desire to be parents, we must first master the role of a child.

Let me give you an example of how God rewards us. God grants us His favor by nature of our relationship with Him. Before I got married, I prayed for a godly man. I wanted a man that would love God more than me, so in those tough times, God would show him how to love me.

My fiancée and I were sitting in church one Sunday when the pastor started preaching on tithing. My fiancée, now my husband, leaned over and asked me if I tithed. I proudly said, "I put in twenty dollars every Sunday." Now at that time, my yearly income was fairly average income, so he replied "Twenty dollars!" That's not a tithe, that's a tip. The tithe is ten percent of your income, twenty dollars is nowhere near ten percent of your income. I said, "There is no way I can pay that to the church every two weeks, that is way too much," He quietly said to me, "We will be tithing our money once we get married, so you better get used to it now."

I really didn't know what he meant at the time, but he quickly let me know. Before we got married, he encouraged me to start tithing and he reminded me of the scriptures on tithing like the one in *Malachi 3:8 which says, "Will a man rob God? Yet you are robbing Me! But you say, How have we robbed You? In tithes and offerings."*

I felt ashamed. There is an old saying, "Be careful what you pray for, you might just get it." Well, I prayed for a godly man, and I got one. So we looked at my income and he determined what 10% of my salary would be. I was absolutely shocked that it was so much! I could not believe it. I said, "I want to obey, but I don't know how I can afford to pay that much." He said, "Don't worry you will." We got married and started tithing just as he said we would. I kept quiet because I wanted to please God. Also, I could see this was an argument that my husband was not backing down from.

Our first year together, we watched God reward us for our faith in tithing. Almost every month, we'd find an extra $100 or $200 dollars in our checking account. Now, I know what many of you are thinking reading this book, obviously there was a mistake or error in the checkbook. But before you continue that line of thinking, let me tell you that my husband balances the checkbook to the penny! If the balance is not correct with the bank's assessment, he will check it over and over until he finds the mistake. He wants all of the debits and credits to balance. For the first three years of our marriage, there were many occasions where Steven tried to balance the checkbook, always checking with the bank to understand an extra $100 or $200 dollar discrepancy. Every time it was to no avail. There was no bank error and no error on his part, it was God's reward to us. Steven would just highlight the extra money and add a little note to the line item saying, "Thank You God." The Bible says in Matthew 25:21, *"Well done, good and faithful servant. You were faithful with a few things, I will put in charge of many things…"* You might think a $100 or $200 is not a lot, but when you don't have a lot and are newly married, acquiring each others bills, trust me, every bit helps.

Seed Time/Harvest Time Principle:

In this area, sow a seed into a child's life that has succeeded in accomplishing a task. Find a child who needs some encouragement and reward him/her. Everyone wants to feel like they are doing a good job. It's doesn't have to be anything expensive, just give him a small token to let him know you are proud of him. We never know how something like this can change a child's life.

III

The Daughter's Arrival
Into Destiny

13

Driven to Dream

Kim is now experiencing deep rooted joy because she is charged with faith. Consistently, she's been talking and walking with God and has reached a point of contentment with herself, her body, her husband and most importantly, her God. She is holding on to God and knows that He is holding on to her. This newfound peace has caused her to reevaluate everything in her life. She no longer sees problems as problems, but now sees them as opportunities for God to show up with His power and grace to overcome the impossible. Kim is functioning on faith in God, but also with the faith of God.

Instead of charting her ovulation and taking the infertility treatments, she now focuses on enjoying God, life and her husband. Spontaneity has returned to her marriage. Knowing that she's heard from heaven, she trusts that God will bless her womb. She doesn't know when the blessing will come, but she's Okay with that because she knows God's word is true. So she continues to wait with a tranquil spirit.

Through her increased relationship with Him, Kim has learned that God shows her that enemies such as doubt and deception don't have a place in her life when He is placed first in her heart. Everything she's been through was all in preparation for this time of contentment. Now, she's not only walking in faith, she's walking with a spirit of expectancy. She expects God to answer, but recognizes that He is sovereign and only He decides when she will have a baby. Still she waits, but waiting has turned into time for preparation, as she clips coupons for diapers and formula.

Today, something is very wrong and she is not sure what it is. She feels lethargic, almost like her body has hit rock bottom. It's not quite time for her cycle, so what could be making her feel this way? Her stomach feels like it has stiffened at the very bottom. The thought crosses her mind, "Maybe I am pregnant?" However, that idea is quickly dismissed because this feeling is nothing like the feeling she had before. In fact, this feeling is totally opposite. After praying so hard for a baby, Kim is now concerned about her age and whether her parents would live long enough to see their grandchild grow up. Has this excess anxiety caused her to experience some other type of illness. All she ever wanted was a baby and to have a family and now what has she done. A week or two go by and she still feels awful. Finally, it's time for her period and she thinks maybe that will flush her system and cause her body to feel better. After more days, now her cycle is officially late. Again, she does not get excited because her cycle has been late many times before. She's sure that it will show up in a couple of days. For a moment, she begins imagining that maybe she is pregnant. How would she tell her husband who has been waiting for years as well?

Well, instead of planning a nice dinner or telling him in the baby aisle of a store, she just mentions it to him in passing. As suspected, he's elated; however, she cautions him that she has not taken a pregnancy test and wants to wait a little longer to make sure her cycle does not start. She doesn't want his hopes up because she has been late before; she has taken this test many times and it has been negative many times. Of course, every day he wants to take the test, until finally she gives in and they take the test. "IT"S POSITIVE!!!! I AM PREGNANT!!!!!" Kim wakes up from her nap and realizes that she slept longer than she had intended. She feels disoriented because she just had her dream come true. Only, then she wakes up, it was truly just a dream; but, it seemed so real; so she really wasn't sure if she was dreaming or not. Her faith is charged even more because she knows she was driven to dream this dream. She can't wait to see when God is going to make her dreams come true. As she pauses, she begins to analyze the trial of infertility and the three lessons she learned: the first lesson was in the area of peace. Since the initial ordeal of infertility, Kim wrestled with living in peace. Not knowing when or if she would ever become pregnant kept her in a sea of imbalance. From month to month and year to year, she functioned in turmoil. It was as if she constantly held her breath that maybe this time, this month, this year, God would answer the prayer that she so desperately needed answered. Until she came to the realization that real peace did not involve whether or not she gave birth to a child; real peace involved God.

Focusing on Him and realizing that He, and He alone, provides the kind of peace that sustains you during your waiting period. Understanding and applying this concept is the key to our whole being. Without peace in your life you function in turmoil, disarray and uncertainty. Peace is a gift from God and we should never function in this life without it. *Ephesians 2:14 states, "For He Himself is our peace…"* Let me explain in further detail, *peace through God* provides the *peace of God* and the *peace of God* gives us the *peace with God*. *Colossians 1:20 states, "For it was the Father's good pleasure for all the fullness to dwell in Him, and through Him to reconcile all things to Himself, having made peace through the blood of His cross; through Him…."* God provides for us to have peace through Him. When Jesus Christ died on the cross for our sins, He also provided us with peace through Him. Without Jesus' sacrifice, we could never have or know everlasting peace. By accepting His sacrifice, we have peace through Him. Only because He graciously gave Himself for us, can we have this peace. Permanent peace with God cannot abide without God.

You may think, "Well, I'm already at peace with myself." However, if it is not based on the foundation of Christ, it is considered temporary peace. Temporary peace is when you experience moments of bliss that are not long lasting. This leads us to a discussion of the peace of God. For example, you take a vacation for a week to a beautiful Caribbean island. You allow yourself to forget about your problems, your job, the bills etc. For that week, you bask in the sun, enjoying great food and fun events; you feel at peace.

As soon as you board the plane back home, you remember the problems you left that now must be addressed. You think about the work that is stacked on your desk as well the stressful conversations you need to have with your boss. Lastly, you think about your bills, possibly how you will pay for this island vacation. Suddenly, these thoughts overshadow your mind and you are thrust back into worry and anxiety. Your peace on the island was merely a moment of bliss, not a long lasting state of being. *John 14:27 states, "Peace I leave with you; my peace I give to you; not as the world gives do I give to you. Do not let your heart be troubled nor let it be fearful."* The world provides a temporary peace in that is not long lasting. When you have God's peace, you don't have to be on an island for complete relaxation and peace. You can be in a busy airport with hordes of people complaining about their flight delays and still maintain a spirit of peace.

You might say "Well, that wouldn't really stress me out." Okay, let me give you another example closer to home. You've missed your period and you're elated because this has never happened before. You take a pregnancy test and the test shows positive. You contact your doctor and he advises that you come in for an exam. You go in and find out that you are really pregnant. You are so happy and you begin sharing your good news with others.

Time goes by and it's time for another check-up. This time, you'll get to hear the baby's heartbeat, but, the doctor can't find the heartbeat. They perform a vaginal sonogram and the sack is there, but it is empty. There is no baby. Do you have the peace of God? Yes, you are hurt and confused, but somewhere in your despair you remember that God will sustain you through any storm. Don't get me wrong, this would cause anyone to pause—even out of pure shock; but, if you're walking with the peace of God, you will respond differently because this is another opportunity for God to show up on your behalf. *Philippians 4:7 states "And the peace of god which surpasses all comprehension will guard your hearts and your minds in Christ Jesus."*

This brings us to the peace with God. Once you have the peace of God, then you are at peace with God. Let me explain further, peace with God means that you are not angry and/or you are not holding a grudge against God for a miscarriage or for not answering your prayers as quickly as you would have thought He would. Instead of this stance, you tap into your faith and rely on that faith to sustain you through whatever storm you are going through. God sees your effort and rewards you. *Romans 5:1 states, "Therefore having been justified by faith, we have peace with God through our Lord Jesus Christ."* Verse five further states, *"....and hope does not disappoint because the love of God has been poured out within our hearts through the Holy Spirit who was given to us."* When you are at peace with God, this allows Him to show you some things that perhaps you didn't know about yourself. He even goes further by pouring His love in our hearts which heals all our hurts, disappointments and upsets.

How wonderful is He? He takes the time to make sure that His grace and peace fill us with so much more than we could ever imagine.

The second lesson Kim learned was in the area of contentment. Now we have touched upon contentment a little in the earlier chapters, but we have not fully dissected this concept. Contentment means to be satisfied with your current situation regardless of the present external circumstances. You might be thinking to yourself, but how do I get there? My feelings are in direct contradiction with contentment.

There are (4) four steps to arriving at contentment. The first step is to identify the problem. The problem is "I want to have a baby and as of yet, my body and my mind are not cooperating." When you acknowledge the problem, you do two things: 1) you admit that there is something that you are unhappy with and you want it to be solved and 2) you acknowledge that you are unable or ill-equipped to handle it alone and you need help. Let's face it, if you could handle it yourself, the problem would no longer be a problem; it would be fixed.

The next step is to face the reality of the problem. In this example, you might say, "I have tried to have a baby for years and nothing is happening and because of this I am frustrated. I want to know when I am going to have a baby." Steps 1 and 2 are based on your thoughts and feelings; however Step 3 involves submitting that problem and the reality of it to God.

Well Okay, how do I do that? Start by memorizing *Galatians 2:20 which states, "I have been crucified with Christ and it is no longer I who live, but Christ lives in me; and the life which I now live in the flesh I live by faith in the Son of God, who loved me and gave Himself up for me."* This verse takes the focus off of you and your circumstances and places the focus on God and what He did for you. In essence, you are exchanging your will for His will. Your response might be, "Yes I want to have a baby, but I want only what God wants for me. He may not want to bless me with a child right now, because He wants my attention focused elsewhere." Or maybe you need to spend some time completely focused on Him or maybe He has a child He wants you to adopt. I don't know what God's will is for your life; all I know is that God does everything for a reason. We may not always understand it, but we must have peace and contentment with Him and in Him because He is sovereign and there is nothing we can do about why He does certain things in our lives. *John 3:30 states, "He must increase, but I must decrease."* We have to stop focusing on what we want and focus on what He wants—it's not about us or our agenda.

Stop thinking to yourself, "If I don't have a baby soon, I'm going to be too old." God is the Father of time, not man. Man may say, "By this age, you must have a child or it's too risky," Don't get caught up on what man says. God created man and God does not function according to man's time. God is only concerned about what He says regarding time and the timing of your blessing.

This leads to Step 4, acknowledging the sovereignty of God while you await your blessing. *Colossians 1:16 states, "For by Him all things were created....... all things have been created through Him and for Him."* So regardless of what we think regarding our fertility, God is in charge. Stop thinking, "If I hadn't had an abortion, or maybe I should have had those fibroid tumors removed earlier, then I would be pregnant. You are not pregnant because God has not allowed you to be pregnant and give birth to a child. It's not the physical or emotional status, it is God's status. Again, He has a reason for everything He does. That's why *Matthew 6:33* states, *"Seek first the kingdom of God and His righteousness and all these things will be added to you."* We need to understand, that's how God works. Once we acknowledge His sovereignty and place our faith in Him, then we receive blessing; but, you cannot place sovereignty in your doctor, your husband or what some friend told you to do to get pregnant. You have to go to God, first.

It was only after following these steps that I arrived at contentment. I told God on more then one occasion, "If you never bless my womb, I will still praise you." After awhile, I grew content in my stance with God. I knew that He was sovereign and He could do anything; it was just a matter of when. When I saw pregnant women, I was happy for them because I focused on the day that God would bless me as well. In the stores, baby clothes and baby items looked different to me. No longer was I looking out of sadness or anger, but out of intrigue as to what items God would bless me to use when my little bundle arrived. I walked in an air of contentment, seeing others celebrating and realizing that my day was on its way. God had given me peace and contentment, which in turn was building my faith in Him and His promises for me.

The third lesson Kim learned was in the area of faith. *Hebrews 11:1*, states, *"Now faith is the assurance of things hoped for, but the evidence of things not seen."* This means, even when you cannot see your blessing on the horizon, you know it's coming, so you wait for it to show up any moment. It's been said, "Faith is when you act like God is telling the truth." Many say they have faith, but their actions speak otherwise.

Let me tell you a story that comes from Luke Chapter 1. This story involves a priest named Zacharias and his wife Elizabeth. This couple was older and Elizabeth was barren. Both had a desire to have a child and the Bible says they were righteous in the sight of God. One day, Zacharias was performing his priestly duties in the temple when an angel appeared and told him that he would have a son and his name would be John. Zacharias asked a disturbing question, "How will I know this for certain?"

The angel responded, *"…behold you shall be silent and unable to speak until the day when these things take place, because you did not believe my words, which will be fulfilled in their proper time."* There are consequences to not having faith in what God has said. For Zacharias, it was temporarily muteness due to his unbelief.

Make sure that your faith is in God and that you believe what He says He will do. *Hebrews 11:6* states, *"without faith, it is impossible to please God."* Without faith, God is not pleased with us and does not bless us with the desires of our heart. We must believe in Him and what He says. Faith and prayer provide access to God. We need to exercise both of these tools in order to receive the blessing that God has in store for us.

As I went about my daily chores, my husband kept asking me, "How are you feeling?" For which I answered, "Fine." It was a Saturday, and of course, we had a ton of errands to run, so I continued with all my activities. Kindly, my husband replied, "Maybe you should rest. I can do some of the errands for you." I had to ask him, "Why are you being so nice to me? Not that you are not nice, but you seem to be extra nice today." And he said, "Why wouldn't I? You're pregnant and I want you to get all the rest you need. We're not going to rush around like usual, we're taking it easy." "What did you say?"

He said, "Remember, we took the test yesterday and it was positive."

Now, I must really be tripping. I knew that I had dreamed that, but this almost seemed real…in fact, it was real! I listened again to what he was saying. I had taken the test yesterday and it was positive. My God, why did I think I was dreaming?

Sometimes, God can bless us and we are too scared to believe the blessing. You see, I blocked it out as though it was a dream. I believed in God and I believed in His power, but I was completely overwhelmed when it finally did happen. Don't allow yourself to believe that it is going to happen and then when it does you want to back away because it's too real, unbelievable. Know this, faith in God does work, His promises are true and dreams do come true.

When you build your faith to the place where you can truly believe that it's going to happen, sometimes it knocks you over when it actually does happen. It's there, it's real and it's unbelievable. I encourage you to be driven to dream.

14

Defeating Difficulty

Jeremiah 32:27—Behold, I am the Lord, the God of all flesh, is anything too difficult for Me?

We walked into the doctor's office elated knowing that God had finally answered our prayers. However, we left extremely cautious. Because of my age, prior miscarriages, fibroid tumors and endometriosis, I was considered a high risk pregnancy. My doctor fully explained the danger signs and things about which to be concerned. He immediately started me on a medication called progesterone. This medication is used to prevent a miscarriage and increase the lining of the uterus. I was told it was not harmful to the baby or to me, but it was important that I take the medication everyday until the end of the first trimester. While I thought this was odd, no one else I knew had to take medication. I decided I would do whatever I needed to do to make sure my baby made it here safely.

As we drove home, I began to think about the lining of my uterus. The lining had to be thickened in order for a miscarriage not to occur and for my baby to survive. How do you make something thick? I suppose by placing layers on top of layers until the multitude of layers makes it thick. Progesterone would add layers onto the lining of my uterus causing it to withstand the weight of a fetus. Then it dawned on me, I needed to make my faith thick. Yes, I had great faith before I arrived to this point, but God moving me into another dimension of faith. He wanted me to layer my faith to make it that much stronger. I had "walked in faith" up to this point, but now I was faced with a "faith walk." It is hard to "walk in faith", but it's even more difficult to "faith walk".

Let me explain the difference. "Walking in faith" is praying and believing that God is going to answer your prayers simply because He has the power to do it. Regardless of what comes your way, you are patiently expecting God to do the supernatural in your physical and emotional body. You know what God's Word says regarding conception, pregnancy and birth and you are just waiting for God to bless you. While "walking in faith," you have conquered fear in this area and you are at peace and content with your present circumstances. Now, walking the "faith walk" is totally different because this walk means that God has answered your prayers, you have conceived and everything looks great until complications and/or obstacles occur. For me, both were challenging.

I had to *thicken my faith* in God because fear crept back into my psyche. I thought, "What if I take the medicine and it doesn't work? What if I started taking it and it was already too late because my lining was too thin? Would the medicine harm my baby even though the doctor said it would not?" All sorts of thoughts ran rampant in my head. I had to gain control and focus on thickening my faith.

During my faith walk, I found two ways to accomplish this: 1) praying in faith and 2) practicing faith. I began by praying in faith that God would hold my lining together, thicken it and make it stronger than ever. I started with *1 Peter 4:8*, which states, *"Therefore be of sound mind and sober spirit for the purpose of prayer."* I followed this by *1 Peter 5:7* which states, *"Casting all your anxiety on Him because He cares for you."* I had to examine what I feared. I wanted God to bless my womb and allow me to conceive and He had that. But instead of greatly rejoicing, I was fearful of the future. Praying in faith and believing in God was the only thing that got me through this period. I realized that you cannot pray and worry simultaneously; you can do one or the other, but not both. Praying and worrying are two opposites. The Bible says *in 1 John 4:18, "There is no fear in love; but perfect love casts out fear, because fear involves punishment, and the one who fears is not perfected in love."* I figured I couldn't disappoint God after all He had answered my prayers; why was I worried? I knew God loved me and wanted to give me His best. I had to stand firm in my faith.

As a result of praying in faith, I began practicing faith. If I thought I felt a twinge in my abdomen, I just prayed and it left. I found that some of the things I felt, I had only imagined. I remembered reading in *James 5:16, "The fervent prayers of the righteous availed much."* So, I finally began to walk in this blessing and enjoy it. My advice is that you thicken your faith even before God opens your womb and drops off your blessing. While you're praying to God and asking Him to do the miraculous, thicken your faith. And if you see your cycle on a month that you believed you conceived, don't get upset and say, "Here it is again, I hate when this happens." Instead, thicken your faith by saying, "Well, maybe I'm not pregnant this month, but God, I know you're going to do this. I'm not giving up." Always know that your blessing is closer than you think.

At the beginning of my fourth month, I noticed that I was experiencing severe pain in my abdomen. I read pregnancy books and talked to friends that told me it was just my body stretching, but I knew in my spirit, it was much more. My husband and I went to the doctor and I told him about the pain. He explained that as my body stretched I would feel some discomfort. I explained to him that this was not "discomfort," but excruciating pain. He was concerned and ordered the technician to perform a sonogram. As the technician moved the instrument over my body, she called my doctor into the room. We couldn't tell from the screen what was wrong, but he came in and looked at the screen. He told us that a tumor was growing on the opposite side from the baby. Panic and fear gripped both me and my husband. My first miscarriage was caused by a tumor inside competing with our baby and that time, the tumor won.

Just imagine our shock and disappointment. Here we were facing the same obstacle as three years before, the same obstacle that has caused so much hurt, so much pain. We didn't know what to say or think, feeling like our dreams were dashed. The doctor gave us several possibilities. He said that many times the tumor, continues to grow during pregnancy and currently it was the size of a quarter. He told us that if the tumor grows faster than the baby, it would cause us to miscarry again. The other scenario he mentioned was the possibility of taking the baby at around the sixth or seventh month. That is, if the baby was still growing in competition with the tumor. My husband asked if there was a chance that the tumor could shrink or dissolve. The doctor said it could, but it is not likely. He further stated that with each visit, I would need to have a sonogram to determine the size and growth of the tumor.

We left the doctors office and headed home. I was silent most of the way, but my husband was not. He kept reassuring me that God would not bring us this far and leave us. He repeated to me words of faith and told me we were not giving up on God. I heard him, and I knew he was right. This obstacle was just another test, another opportunity for God to show Himself strong. God had thickened our faith, and now He was _stretching and growing our faith_. I needed to hear from God in a whole new way and He led me to _Hebrews 12:1-3, "Lay aside every encumbrance and the sin that so easily entangles us, and let us run with endurance the race that is set before us, fixing our eyes on Jesus, the author and perfecter of our faith."_ I couldn't allow fear and anxiety to come back to my mind or cause me to take my eyes off Christ.

There is a story in Matthew 14:28 where Peter was walking on the water to Jesus? As long as Peter focused on Jesus standing before him on the water, he was able to walk on water. The minute Peter took his eyes off Jesus and focused on the wind and the waves, he began to sink. Like Peter, when I took my eyes off of God and focused on the tumor inside, I began to sink. I had to go back and pray in faith. Even more I had to practice my faith.

The doctor prescribed hydrocodeine for the pain I was experiencing. Again, he told me the medication would not harm the baby. I tried not to take the medication, but the pain became so bad that I felt like I didn't have a choice. I took one pill and felt like I was out of my head. I was light headed and couldn't focus on anything. I could only imagine what my baby was experiencing. The experience of the first pill caused me not to take another pill. I endured the pain, which at times seemed unbearable. One morning, my husband woke up and decided that he would pray and lay hands on my abdomen asking God to shrink and dissolve the tumor. At this point, my faith was little. Experiencing pain day in and day out without medication had drained my energy and my faith. I was fatigued beyond belief. I heard my husband's prayer and hoped that God would answer quickly, but I was so tired. Tired of fighting, tired of praying and tired of hurting. I wanted to have my baby, but I wanted the pain to end. I had missed several days from work; I felt as though I was no good to anyone. I was functioning in a cloud, not sure of today and not sure of tomorrow, only sure of God.

As my husband prayed, I felt heat generating from his hands on my abdomen. At first, I moved his hands away, but he continued praying and laying his hands on me. There was so much heat from his hands until I felt that God was healing me through his hands. It was hard to explain, but very powerful.

That day, I did not experience any pain. The next day, the pain returned, but with less intensity. I knew something was going on, but I didn't know what.

I was reminded of the woman in Matthew 9:20 that had the issue of a never-ending flow of blood. She simply touched the hem of Jesus' garment and she was healed of her infirmity, immediately. Now don't get me wrong, my husband is not God, nor do I compare him to God, but I do believe that God sends His power to us by way of the Holy Spirit and allows us to disseminate His power to others. My faith had been shaken, but God was restoring it daily. The pain in my abdomen was becoming less everyday.

On my next doctor's appointment, as expected, my doctor asked for another sonogram. My husband and I waited as the technician performed the test. She immediately, called the doctor again to come in and look at the screen. He came in, looked at the screen and asked the technician to move the instrument to the other side. She moved the instrument and the screen looked the same. The doctor said, "No, that's not right. Look again." Again, she performed as instructed and the result was still the same. The doctor told us that they could not find the tumor, but that it had probably moved and was hiding. He told us not to get too excited because the tumor was probably still there. He just couldn't find it. He said that he would perform another sonogram the next month. It was at this point that I informed him that I had stopped taking the medication a couple of weeks earlier and the pain was gone. Steven and I were praising Jesus because we knew the tumor had not moved—it was gone.

Things progressed pretty well for awhile. That is, until I reached my sixth month of pregnancy. It all started while I was at work when I suddenly felt pain my abdomen. I immediately knew that something was wrong. I told my assistant and she suggested that we call the paramedics to check me out. They arrived shortly after we called, determined that I was having contractions and rushed me to the hospital. Arriving at the hospital, the emergency nurses immediately started an IV as I waited for the contractions to stop and looked for my husband to arrive. After performing many tests, they advised me that I was dehydrated, causing my body to be forced into labor. As I laid there, my husband arrived and I explained to him what they told me. He took my hand and we prayed for God to take care of me and our baby.

Hours passed and doctors and nurses continued to monitor my contractions. Although, I was scared, something in me told me that God was going to restore my health as well as the health of our baby. The contractions slowed and became less and less noticeable until I was finally out of the woods. God had restored me by pouring living water in me to replace the water that was poured out of me. Yet once again, we were so grateful and exceedingly thankful for God's grace.

15

Destiny—Children of the Promise

Romans 9:8—It is not the children of the flesh who are children of God, but the children of the promise are regarded as descendents.

Kim sighs and says, "Well, today is the day." One week overdue, Kim is admitted into the hospital and is assigned a room. The IVs and other tubing are hooked up to her cervix and arm. Her doctor performed a new balloon procedure where he attached a weight to gently pull the cervix, causing it to dilate slowly. It was uncomfortable, but necessary.

Kim had been experiencing contractions on and off, but labor did not mature. It took six hours before her cervix dilated after contractions first began. As one might imagine, the contractions then came with a vengeance. Kim was given an epidural for the pain. It was the part she dreaded more than anything else because they inserted a long needle near an area of the spine. However, as the pain became increasingly worse, Kim did not concern herself with the size of the needle nor its intended destination. She just wanted the pain to end.

After several hours of pushing, then resting and then pushing again, the nurse touched the area surrounding the baby's head and surprisingly Kim screamed. She could feel everything! The pain had come back with great intensity. It was unbearable. After about a half-hour, the anesthesiologist was paged. He needed to double-check the procedure that had been performed earlier that evening. He couldn't believe that she was able to feel anything. He raised her up and checked the epidural and found blood in the line. Apparently, the epidural was not inserted correctly. The doctor was visibly frustrated and asked why they never noticed the blood in the line. A second epidural was inserted and she was encouraged to get some rest. "We'll try again in a few hours."

The doctor came in early that morning and informed Kim and Steven that they needed to have the baby out in an hour or else he would have to perform an emergency c-section. He didn't believe that Kim would be able to push the baby through, and he was concerned because the baby's heart rate had started to drop. Kim began to push, but she also started praying. Instantly, God answered. After a few short minutes of pushing, Kim delivered a healthy, 8 lb. 12 oz. baby girl. At 21.5 inches in length, she was a very big baby.

God had done the miraculous. This miracle was a visible sign to me that God can do anything. There is nothing too hard for Him. It has been six years since the start of writing this book, and as I sit here finishing this final chapter, I am reminded of my years of struggle with infertility. Through it all, I remain thankful for this trial. It's easy to want to rush through any trial to arrive on the other side, but without going through the process, we can miss out on the blessings that can only be taught in the storm. I have learned so much about God, about myself and about the life-long valuable lessons He so patiently taught me.

You see, it was in this process, where God transformed me into a joyful mother. By His example of parenting and teaching the lessons He wanted me to learn: peace, contentment and faith, He transformed my mind and my body to be aligned with His will. God took what appeared to be the impossible and made it possible. He is a good God! Now, my prayer is that whatever God is teaching you, that you will go through the process with an open mind and open heart. Be open to what He wants to teach you, open to His will and His timing for your life. And realize, no matter what your situation is: He and He alone has the power to transform you into a joyful mother.

About the Author

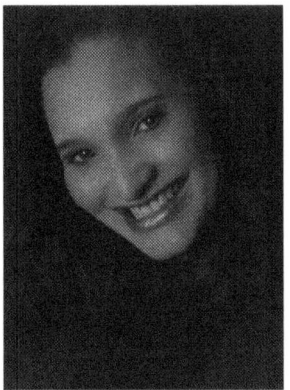

Kimberly Webb is intimately familiar with infertility, suffering through many surgeries to correct fibroid tumors, irregular periods, endometriosis, miscarriages as well as a tubal pregnancy. She has first-hand experience with the physical pain and emotional strain these circumstances cause. However, she has endured the struggles of infertility and has learned God's process of transforming infertile women into joyful mothers. This is what He did with her in the years prior to the birth of her daughter. As an accomplished speaker, Kim is a powerful orator who leaves an indelible mark on all those who come in contact with her—regularly speaking to women on issues concerning infertility, self identity and marriage. Additionally, Kim has more than five years of experience as a Christian pre-marital and marital counselor. Mrs. Webb is a graduate from Howard University with a B.A. in Political Science and a Juris Doctorate of Law degree from Texas Wesleyan University. Kim and her husband reside in Carrollton, Texas with their daughter.

978-0-595-39449-4
0-595-39449-3

www.ingramcontent.com/pod-product-compliance
Lightning Source LLC
Chambersburg PA
CBHW051433280526
45785CB00003B/1277